The Iceberg

The Iceberg

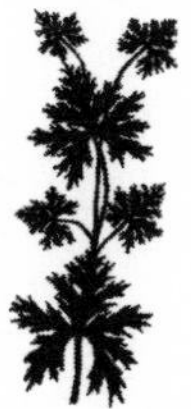

MARION COUTTS

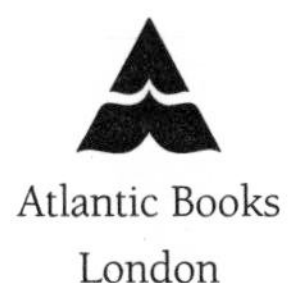

Atlantic Books
London

Published in hardback in Great Britain in 2014 by Atlantic Books,
an imprint of Atlantic Books Ltd.

10 9 8 7 6 5 4 3 2

A CIP catalogue record for this book is available from the British Library.

Hardback ISBN: 9781782393504
E-book ISBN: 9781782393511

Printed and bound by CPI Group (UK) Ltd, Croydon, CR0 4YY

Atlantic Books
An Imprint of Atlantic Books Ltd
Ormond House
26–27 Boswell Street
London
WC1N 3JZ

www.atlantic-books.co.uk

Let It Go

It is this deep blankness is the real thing strange.
The more things happen to you the more you can't
Tell or remember even what they were.
The contradictions cover such a range.
The talk would talk and go so far aslant.
You don't want madhouse and the whole thing there.

– William Empson

SECTION I

1.1

A book about the future must be written in advance. Later I won't have the energy to speak. So I will do it now.

The others are near. I can touch them, call them to me and they are here. We are all here, Tom, my husband, and Ev, our child. Tom is his real name and Ev is not really called Ev but Ev means him. He is eighteen months old and still so fluid that to identify him is futile. We will all be changed by this. He the most.

The home is the arena for our tri-part drama: the set for everything that occurs in the main. We go out, in fact all the time, yet this is where we are most relaxed. This is the place where you will find us most ourselves.

Something has happened. A piece of news. We have had a diagnosis that has the status of an event. The news makes a rupture with what went before: clean, complete and total save in one respect. It seems that after the event, the decision we make is to remain. Our unit stands. This alone will not save us but whenever we look, it is the case. The decision is joint and tacit and I am surprised to realise this. Though we talked about countless things – talk is all we ever do – we did not address it directly. So not a decision then, more a mode, arrived at together.

The news is given verbally. We learn something. We are mortal. You might say you know this but you don't. The news falls neatly between one moment and another. You would not think there was a gap for such a thing. You would not think there was room. The threat has two aspects: a current fact and an obscure outcome – the manifestation of the fact. The first is immediate and the second talks of duration. The fact has coherent force and nothing, no person or thought or thing, escapes its shift. It is as if a new physical law has been described for us bespoke: absolute as all the others are, yet terrifyingly casual. It is a law of perception. It says, *You will lose everything that catches your eye.* Under this illumination there is no downtime and no off-gaze. For its duration, looking can never be idle. Seeing is active: it is an action like aiming or hitting.

Yet afterwards – more strangeness – we carry on in many ways as before, but crosswise to what might be expected, we are not plunged into night. It is still day, but the light is unnatural. The glare on daily life is blinding. Everything is equally illumined, without shade.

These are early days. Our house becomes porous. I am high and bleached and whited out. We are air and the walls are air. On hearing the news, our instinct is to tell it. Once known it cannot be unlearned; once told, not rescinded. So we start to speak, and the family, we three, are dissolved in fluid and drunk up by others. People appear, they come and go. They are always to hand. Ev is in his element and we are in ours. As I say, these are early days. Maybe it will always be like this.

1.2

It is Ev's first day at the childminder's. I arrive at nine, anxious and grave and trying not to show it. This is our first official separation. The mother of one is a volatile mix of niche knowledge and inexperience. I am a zealot. I have rolls of data to proclaim about his protocols: his beaker, when he likes to nap, his poo, his play, his pleasures, the snacks that are allowed and the snacks that are forbidden. I am not going to let anything stop me.

The childminder lives around the corner. She is much younger than me and canny. She has heard all this before. She knows to be patient and let me play myself out. When I am done, she will take the child. I eye her up and scan the house for flaws as I recite my speech. *Is that a very sharp edge? That stair-gate looks shaky. The kitchen could be tidier. I know she has dogs; where are they? Why am I putting him in a house with dogs?* We both understand that my rhetoric is symbolic, the words a verse-chorus lament to mark the movement of the child out of my orbit and into another: out of the home and into the world.

In mid-song I am interrupted. Tom arrives. I am surprised to see him and pleased. Lately we have been seriously upended. A week ago, while we were staying at the house of friends, he had a fit. We don't know why. He never had one before and the shock took us straight into hospital in the night. In the wake of this we have been unnerved, though slowly calming as he has been fine since and anyway, there is Ev to think about. Soon we expect some test results from the hospital. I imagine a letter about high blood pressure or diet, some readily managed condition, normal, nothing beyond us, nothing outwith the stretch of mid-life or span of circumstance. If you were to ask me, that's what I would say. But really I am not imagining anything. I am thinking about Ev.

Tom greets me directly and takes my sleeve, pulling Ev and me out of the yard away from the toys and into the street. It's good he is here. He recognises the importance of my mission and is come in solidarity to support me. I am an airship on its maiden voyage packed with mother adrenalin. The band is playing. Ascent is the most dangerous moment. I have already left the ground, my skin taut with the child and his real and imagined needs. The three of us cluster a couple of doors down alongside a white house with a low lilac wall. Number 36. Alpines, succulents and tiny sedum rooted in the shallowest scattering of earth are planted in gaps along its brickwork. Ev wriggles in my arms and I am still talking. *Ev is so relaxed. He likes her. He will be happy here.* Tom stops me. He says he has had a phone call. He has a brain tumour. It is very likely malignant.

Did I understand it before I heard it or did he finish the sentence before I understood? Conflagration: my ship is exploded. A fireball. Tears fall as burning fuel. There is no time for anything to be saved. There is no time for anything to sink in. There is no time. The word is the deed. The deed is done before knowledge can release its meaning. It is the quickest poison.

I am crushing Ev and my crying escalates. When did it start – before, or after? I don't understand. It seems I was crying before I heard it. Ev starts to wail and this brings the childminder on to the street and frightens the other child in her care, Ev's new friend-in-waiting. He runs to the gate and looks at us blankly. *What are they doing?* The ceremony is over. Ev's rite of passage is abandoned. Tom gives him into the arms of a stranger and we flee.

Did I go back and pick him up at four? I don't remember how he came home but somehow at the end of the day he is back with us. By his face I see he is content in the new world he has inherited so precipitately: dogs, children, a yard outside to play in, plastic toys stained with rain. It is strange. He is entirely unblemished. Not a mark on him. He is unharmed, happy even. When we left the house that morning we were blithe. We were not conscious of death. We knew it existed, but not for us.

That day, the first near-coherent thing I say after many hours is to Tom. *I cannot lose all of you to all of him. I will not.*

Right from the start see how I set myself up. Let us see how this thing goes.

1.3

The day of the diagnosis delivered by phone we abandon Ev and start walking. Impact has fused us and made us mutual. We are a four-legged creature and we operate manually. Our instinct is to keep in motion. We head south. We talk, but we don't look at anything. The suburbs are good for this kind of inattentiveness. This is what they are for.

After some hours we arrive at Dulwich Picture Gallery. We did not aim to come here and I don't know where else we have been. But now that we are here, Tom needs to look at a painting. When the phone call came he was in the middle of something and there is a picture he wants to look at. Though we both try to recall it, we never again remember which. Perhaps this is the first thing to be noted. That time is continuous. For him the action of looking at a picture is instinctive. It is his work and so familiar, so unremarkable an action that only much later do I wonder at it. There is a particular painting still to be considered. Time hasn't stopped even now. But it spools new. I can feel it – not faster, not slower but with an undertone, a tiny subjective pulse.

Tom's mind is busy. He has a brain tumour but he still has a mind. Where is his mind? Where it was this morning. The brain tumour is in it but the brain tumour is not it. Yesterday and the day before, the day before that, and all the days for however long since, the tumour was already there but we did not know. A thing first hidden in the site of consciousness later becomes knowledge.

We are novices. We have very little information and so repeat what we have. One phrase goes back and forth between us. *The tumour is in the area of speech and language. The tumour is in the area of speech and language*. There is *tumour* and there is *area*. They sound separate, like two entities, one collaged on the other. I do not consider the idea that the tumour might one day take the mind. That thought comes later. Mind trumps tumour. Art trumps everything. Tom goes into the gallery.

In blankness of mind I remain outside. In the garden is a skeletal cypress, blanched sepia and white as if struck by lightning and still erect in its death agony. I stretch out on the grass under this tree and look straight along its length to the point of sky touched by its tip as if it might be showing me something. Some time elapses that I can't describe at all and I am still there when he returns.

Four days later, Ev starts to talk. His sounds have been buffering at meaning for weeks, but now they emerge as his own handiwork and he sets them gently one beside another in lines. I am surprised by this development but everything in this time is unfamiliar: other people, preparing meals, the view outside the window, the first thought in the morning when I wake, Ev's face. It is all something I must get used to, and so his talking is just another thing that has occurred that runs along in parallel to the main.

Children are born into language. They understand the nuances of speech at birth and Ev has been listening to our ceaseless chatter for months in the womb. He has been read to and sung to and laughed at. He knows the pattern of our voices and by its cadence he knows too that something is happening. My face signals it, and the sudden sparks of urgent conversation, the gaps that follow. Ev is spared the violence of knowledge but all the rest he experiences with us. We will learn to be articulate about this together. We are at the beginning.

The impact on our house feels physical. It is as if we have reconfigured the internal architecture or moved the position of the house subtly by degrees with respect to the sun so that the light falls oddly within it. But in the midst of this derangement, Ev's vocabulary as he presents it to us is superlatively normal. He has no words for fear. He says *Daddy* to mean either of us, *kee* for monkey and *Oh no!* at all upsets. *Ssss* serves for snake, the letter S, and any linear thing like a belt or bit of his railway track. He says *click* for light and *sta* for monster, *gakator* for tractor and soon has a small handy clip of words like *digger, apple, spoon, butter, cardi, eye, toast, brush*. *Seem* means machine. He can do *two, three* and *four*.

And in a way that is entirely normal too, we poke him and spur him on. This is what you do with children, goad them for your own enjoyment. *Make a noise like a volcano*, we say. *Make a noise like a firework. Make a noise like a dinosaur*. His eyes are merry. A small, sweet, plosive sound comes from his lips, after each entreaty the same noise, a breath out and a consonant mixed with spit.

1.4

It is my birthday. One week on. We go to a restaurant and take a table in the sun. Radiant September. When they are very young we do not regard our children with much clarity at the best of times and at the table I can scarcely fix Ev in my sight. He is the size of a cat; a thing of gold fur and whitened sunshine. His hands paw and pat the textures of the food as he draws each substance one by one into his mouth: sour, sweet, char, salt, pulp, oil and leaf. It is thrilling to sit with him so grown up. We are here to mark my birthday and something else besides. We make a toast, the least frivolous I will ever make.

To us. To the time that is to come.

When we get home Moses turns up to deliver the sofa. We ordered it from his shop before the diagnosis and here it is after. We can't say no, though it is ridiculous. A second-hand sofa? No, it wasn't us. Regime change. All deals are void. *Keep the money but take it away please*. But here he is manoeuvring it up the stairs before we can do anything about it. We have guests and five of us sit flattened, glasses in hand, on the other two sofas in the room where it is to go. When Moses sets it down, it looks as if it has always been here. We decide that it may stay. More guests can come to sit shiva. It will make room for more sitters.

1.5

To make sense of what is happening, we need to say it aloud. Only then will we hear the news mouthed back by others and reshaped into words – ohs and ahs, expletives, hisses, clicks and long out-breaths. Maybe, coming back to us in this way it will sound different; better, worse, I don't know. Maybe more comprehensible.

So this is what we do. We make an email list of our friends. Concentrating is hard and even remembering who these people are is an effort. We go back to the things we know, the building blocks of our past. Our wedding was nine years ago and at the heart of the list are the wedding guests. We liked these people then and mainly we like them still. Slotted on are new friends met since, lists from subsequent parties, lone figures and friends from more recent, interlocking spheres of the social. We do not edit but add. It is construction work and we are going for solidity: mass, weight and number. Some, who provide their own reason and context or inhabit a singular niche unconnected to the rest by profession or inclination, get left off at first by accident. How on earth did we forget *them*? We are aware that new friends might be made and added, though it feels fraudulent to make friends who know us only in our changed state. We should whisper, *This is not who we really are*. The list is a net: personal, professional, loves and links, close and near, from getting warmer to very hot. Family is here too. Their names are on the computer: itemised, digitised and alphabetical. Now is their hour.

So far only a few people know. The first thing to understand is that endless retelling is overwhelming. It is boring, draining, dispiriting. A tumour is hard to speak of and harder still to hear. I don't have anything else to talk about, but even after the first few attempts, my words sound dulled. It makes a poor recitation. Everyone who hears us wants all the details and the details will be the same: a fit – hospital – a scan – a tumour – cancer – surgery – treatment – uncertainty. The framing of the sequence can be stressed to suit different audiences or the whole might need retelling again from the beginning. Hearing can be veiled by not listening. And our friends and families have their own responses that must be attended to. That is our responsibility. We owe them. We don't want to overburden them or frighten them off. This is our disaster. They are just being called upon to witness.

And where does the stress lie? We don't know. The facts are not many – surgery followed by radiotherapy followed by chemo followed by monitoring. The way the facts fall depends on how you tell it. Is it a story of disaster directly or a version of survival? What route does it take? Is it a story of duration? We don't want to give people the wrong idea but what is the idea? The thing is an ugly knot of accuracy and projection, dead weight and measured hope. Tied up in there somewhere are the statistics. Tom is beginning to describe it. I can barely speak. So together we write them a message in the form of an email.

14 September 2008

Dear Friends

We have some troubling news that you should know. A small tumour has been detected in Tom's brain. It's not known yet whether it is malignant but that is possible. It needs taking out and he'll be operated on in about a week.

We don't know yet what any of this means, in terms of further problems or none, or possible side effects from the operation. It's a very uncertain time for us.

After the first shock, we are strong as we can be. This is largely because Tom is at the moment very well, looks well, is lucid, thoughtful, writing, working, preparing. Ev is fabulous as usual.

At the time of the operation and after, we may need some help. We don't know yet what form this might best take, it could be practical, or just to have our friends in contact, to be phoned up, thought of, emailed, visited.

We will let you know when we have a date for Tom going into hospital.

With love

In the study we bend over the computer, tight under the lamp. Tom presses *Send*. It is serious, this action. By agreeing to its terms and conditions we elect to turn everything pertaining to us a different shade. Once the news has gone out we cannot disavow it or pretend it is not happening. I cannot say I am prepared. I don't have a coherent idea what *Send* means.

I don't have to wait. Messages come back immediately. What were they doing, these people? All hunched over screens so late at night, at home, at work, as if primed and ready to consider Tom's brain? **News, News, News, News:** the word scrolls down in bold text, multiplying in the subject box like a black manifesto printing over and over. Now we are visible. We can be found. The sky has rolled back, revealing the perpetual plains below ceding into darkness. We are isolated and illuminated. From a distance, I can look into our house and see the small family inside it. How easily we may be overrun! How defenceless we are! It is pitiful.

At first, before I understand how it works, I analyse the replies forensically, sifting the words and weighing them. I am searching for signs. It is the most basic superstition, like reading tea-leaves or looking for pictures in a fire. I make instant judgements based on how the words fall and I react in proportion to how dear I hold the friendship. *How much do you love us? Do you know us really? How can you protect us?* I cannot help myself. I might easily hate those who fall short or whose response is lacking. We are in mortal danger and we want to bring our people near, to gather and shield us, stroke us and sing to us. Isolation is death. We will be picked off. That is certain. But email is too crude for divination. The little fonts in stubby lines cannot take it. Words merge and swim about, scarcely readable. Quickly, mercifully the judgements fall away. I have it wrong! This is not about us but about them. We are simply refracted and talked about at second-hand.

There are no rehearsals for these responses. Some have had prior experience in death but whatever they do with us is a first take. All must improvise. Some talk firmly about themselves in long and looping, myopic paragraphs. Some remit their love directly. Some are blessedly, seriously practical. Some are brilliant: full of anecdote and funny. Most are short and this is cleverest. Some come out wrong, missing a connection of word or tone, like an unfinished puzzle or an arrow fired off into a hedge. There are straight-up reminiscences, protestations of love and notes on shock. There are brief, businesslike missives. *Thank you for keeping me informed* – this is perfect and suits very well the sender, like a pair of smart breeches or brogues. Some are hapless. Some do not reply at all and nor do we think less of them. Sending is all and lack of response never deletes them. This is not a group from which you unsubscribe.

We get poems and photos, links to sites, mad advice, offers of dinner, invites, suggestions, jokes, clichés and generosities. Courage in all its forms, liquid and solid, is pressed upon us, pressed and patted, poured and shaped to suit us. But over and above the offers of help and love, precious and determined though they are, is the fact that we are public knowledge. Our signal has been heard. By each response a friend is activated. Our message had a single note. Here is its returning chord.

It goes without saying that I am crying all through this time, except in front of Ev, before whom there seems to be nothing to cry about.

1.6

A new future has been handed to us. Now that it is here, it is impossible to recall what we were expecting before. Ev was born eighteen months ago, so it would have been a lot. But there is no question. The exact texture of past desires cannot be recalled. It is gone.

Ev made more sense to me before as part of a continuum. I study him. He is evident, but the memory of his birth and the circumstances of him coming into being are not. I am reminded that he was born by emergency caesarean. Like a piece of magnetic tape he self-erases neatly. Ever-replacing, refreshing and renewing, he grows older. In the new future, he is coming with us.

Eighteen months later here we are again. It is the same hospital and the schedule of the new future is written on its headed notepaper. Brain surgery as fast as it can be booked, followed by combined chemo- and radiotherapy for the six weeks until Christmas. The chemo is called temozolomide. Six months' more chemo in twenty-eight-day cycles will swallow up the first half of next year, the whole long arc comprising just one round of treatment, one line of attack against the tumour. Each stage will follow the previous one unless we decide to abandon and bail out. It is voluntary. We could do it at any time. But we do not, we sign up.

Tom feels extremely well. Energised by the attention. The surgery is upon us soon, so in the month between diagnosis and operation he and I lose weight. It is best not be overweight for brain surgery and I do it in straight physical alliance. Like giving up smoking, it's easier with two. The kitchen is where we spend much of our time at home and cooking and eating together is both the maintenance and decoration of our days. To differentiate ourselves now would be unthinkable.

I do not have what are called food issues. In normal life I do not weigh myself. I do not have what are called body issues. Mainly I think I look good. I know this might be seen as strange for a western female in her forties but this is one of the points on which I differ from the norm. I don't diet. I don't restrict my intake. I am a size 10 or 12 depending on who is manufacturing. Weight is not something I spend time on.

Tom is much heavier than me. He has two issues around food, or three. He likes it. He is greedy. He eats too much. His diet in the past has been more extreme than mine. In his twenties he would eat Vesta ready-meals. He has eaten at KFC. Of his own volition he would buy a coronation chicken sandwich. I would never do this. His formative food experiences were parlous: an elite public school in the 1970s, forced to eat eggs, both yolk and white, and sauces and slop as was the English way, milk puddings and gammon. Fricassee.

I take charge of the shedding of weight. Here is an area of authority that can be mine. I am focused but not mad and our kitchen diktats are basic and sensible, the ones that everyone really knows. In the kitchen I can expand my theories and believe in their efficacy. Working with colour and smell and taste I will make food that is delicious. In impotence, here is something I can actually do. It is a form of control.

As a new convert I am an extremist and at first my cooking is gross. Leaving fat and pig and seasoning all aside, I make vegetable stews strained of taste and colour. But quickly, it all becomes strangely viable. Small plates, small plates, is the new mantra. I will write a diet book with just this theme. People write books with fewer ideas. It would need padding with cod-science, recipes, edicts, praise, colour photographs and homilies, but basically it would be saying: learn to cook, food you like, not fried, plates 8 cm diameter, not piled high. And don't come back for seconds. On the back of the book there would be an 8 cm dotted line template of a plate to cut out. *Remember – don't pile so high so that the food slides off!* That should make it clear enough. But then I might have to mention cancer.

Everyone should eat off side-plates. Ours are melamine, a set handed down from my grandmother in off-kilter, food-referent colours: mushroom, aubergine and turmeric plus a cracking kingfisher blue. *No salt, no bread, no fat, no dairy, no seconds.* This is written on a Post-it note on the fridge. But neither is the word *No* an absolute. We don't like absolutes. We eat well. The last one, *no seconds,* seems to be key.

We have less than a month before the craniotomy and we get thin fast. People keep coming up to Tom having heard he has cancer and saying *But you look so well*. This makes him laugh. What they mean is, *You are thin! Well* is the euphemism of choice. I head straight for eight stone. One night in the gloom of a restaurant my armpits look like white caverns in the sockets of my dress. I only feel really hungry, dizzy-hungry, once, and that was a clear marker. We must eat. And so we do.

Ev is on another track heading in the opposite direction. He goes at food with intellectual interest and straight joy in taste. It is bonny. If I had known how much pleasure I would get from watching my baby eat I would have thought it an argument for more babies. It is such a treat I can't take my eyes off him and I mask my keenness in case it makes him suspicious that there is something more at stake. So I eat with him, or look out the window or pretend to read the paper. He spoons up lentils, snuffles through tomato sauce with basil and surges his pasta round in it, he dips bread in spinach soup till soup and bread are one and sucks it. He holds broccoli like a cudgel and stuffs one, then two, three, four trees into his mouth. He eats liver! He eats bananas and garlic and stir-fry! We goggle at him. We win and he wins. We all triumph together.

All this differential feeding, fat and lean, exists side by side in the same kitchen. It takes organisation and the organisation is down to me. It comes at a cost: of time, focus, not doing much else apart from the barest bones of my work. But then nothing much else is getting done anyway. Everything is at a cost now. Roasting a sweet potato is priceless. Baking fish in foil is an elevated act. To eat is to partake in the grace. And what could be sweeter than feeding those you love?

1.7

25 September 2008

Dear Friends

Some further news about Tom. He's due to go into hospital on 29 September to have the tumour in his brain removed. He will be in the National Neurological Hospital at Queen Square. The operation will be on the Tuesday. All going well, he should be home by the end of the week.

At the moment nothing can be predicted in terms of recuperation and further treatment. But it's important to us at this time that our friends stay in contact, so please do phone, text, email, visit, and so on, in the coming weeks. If we don't always get back to you at once, don't worry. We hope to see you soon.

With love

Before dawn on the morning of Tom's operation we make a mistake. We have met the surgeon, Mr K, and he is confident, so we are confident. We trust, but we do not know. The consequences are opaque in all this. So we decide to bring Ev into the hospital. As benediction and blessing, all three of us will be present momentarily, like a single stable entity, a stool or tripod. Tom must not go off alone.

It is very early, directly continuous with night. When we arrive, Tom's face has been mapped with marker pen circles and crosses. Thick stickers of green foam dot his cheekbones, temples and forehead. The markers will guide the computer to gauge the entry. The circles are to cross-reference the location of the tumour and point the lie of the head. On the surgeon's table a head is a still-life object, like a cabbage or a clay pot in a painting by Zurbarán, picked out in light against darkness. It must not move.

Tom looks high and mad. He is present but not with us. We cannot make this work or laugh it off as funny face paint. Ev hates face paint, refuses it always. Even without the stickers and the black arrows, Tom's eyes would betray him. Their daylight blue has been tamped into a thicker colour, studded with points of light that glitter in the warm half-dark of the ward. This is brain surgery. We are at altitude and we haven't enough air. Not everyone gets to do this. We are celebrants to this fact. It is strangely festive.

Tom is *Nil by mouth* so as breakfast gets under way we go into a small guest room. A plaque marked with a picture and a date seven years ago names the room in memory of the donor who went this way before. I have brought Ev's yoghurt and fruit mixed in a pot, his pink spoon. Tom tries to feed him but he won't eat. Stupid. Why would he eat? I cannot eat. Tom cannot eat.

It is quiet. No one disturbs us. We could just run away, get the bus and go home or hide out somewhere else. That is the odd thing about hospitals. If you are mobile and have autonomy you can just run. I wonder how many do? If only we could. Belief holds us here; belief in technology, systems, institutions, in the whole apparatus of advanced Western Medicine. We are taking a bet and our belief is that this is the best bet. We stay.

The room is a place for patients to be private and receive guests but there is nowhere to sit and it is full. It has likely been a storeroom since shortly after the plaque went up. Hospitals abhor a void and all good intentions operate against entropy. Excess chairs are piled against the walls and the interior is navigated through stacked tables, wheelchairs, a zimmer frame, a nest of buckets. A noticeboard with nothing on it hangs near the door. Guests seek comfort elsewhere. Here there is none. The lighting is ranged in fierce strips on polystyrene tiles and the walls are two-tone beige separated by a peeling dado. An intense rectangle of back-lit sky at the window affirms that night is on its way into morning. We are getting near.

Ev is frightened. He squirms in Tom's arms. It was a bad idea to bring him. He smells fear on my skin. Is Tom afraid? It doesn't seem so. He is the chosen one, in a solo dream that ends where he does and goes no further. We cannot penetrate it. What are we doing here? Marking the interval between something bad that has happened and something bad that may yet happen. We are always marking things. It is our habit. But we could spend every minute of every day marking and it would never be enough. These daily acknowledgements always have the same aim – like the ill-lit photographs I take today – to achieve permanence, to fix ourselves fast in each other's eyes. With Ev changing from day to day, this is wilful. Still we try.

We are three. The consciousness of one of us is being interrupted. His self-hood is in jeopardy. How will he be? Will he still be mine? What about knowledge of love? That's the main thing. Where does love lie in the brain? Is it marked with a black cross? Will Tom love me and love the boy like he loves us now? If he cannot, how will that affect my love and the boy's love for him?

I don't want to stay though I am afraid of what will happen after we go. Time versus resistance seems an equation for stasis but strangely stasis is not what we have but something else, some other kind of empirical motion. We have brought Ev right into the heart of it and he resists to the full. He knows there is nothing for him here. But some improvised ceremony is called for, and this is it, held among the ramparts of spare furniture. It is now 7 a.m. on a Tuesday in early autumn. Soon I must leave. Soon I must take Ev away. I am not being given a chance to get used to this.

1.8

Tom is having a craniotomy. We who can't be of any assistance here can only lower our eyes and walk the streets like penitents until it is done. After his broken benediction at the hospital I drop Ev at the childminder's. Normality is his best respite. The early light has morphed into a seamless, gunmetal grey that seals the sky from edge to edge. I go back to the hospital without him. Vivien will be my companion but I am destitute, homeless and bodiless. I haven't got this organised, what to do while waiting for the outcome of my husband's brain surgery. There is no protocol. I can do whatever I like.

What I like is to be near. So we decide to stay close, never far from the hospital walls. It is a new attachment. I don't know this area. The neurological hospital is in a part of London I've never had reason to cross, and through a narrow passage off Southampton Row just below the square runs a queer alternative grid of parallel streets. Under different circumstances perhaps I might have discovered it, as it seems to have a range of offerings. The Adult Ed Centre provides courses and big plates of strong dinner. There are gardens for office workers and invalids. Lamb's Conduit Street has a well-heeled mix of bespoke suits, esoteric bag shops, high-end delis, coffee and books. If it were Ev who was sick, I would know the area more than enough. Great Ormond Street is next door.

For something to do I buy a scarf to curb my shivering and hold my coat shut against the wet. I choose it like a lady's favour from a bin of coloured woollens. *This one*, to be worn on the neck in honour of the day. It is a soft, very pale blue. With it laid against my green coat I am the brightest thing in my vision. Everything else is wet ash. We have no agenda but to wait. We try to go to the bookshop to be indoors and have tea but I cannot sit so tame among the other drinkers so we leave. Around the corner is Coram's Fields. I picture Coram as I learned about him at school, a progressive thinker, energetic in breeches, red face, white shirt and wig. The board on the gate says *No adults unaccompanied by minors*. Such a radical idea. We have entered childless but the spirit of Ev is fully with me and no one is here to stop us. This is because it is pouring: a full London pelt. We take cover in the stone gazebo and sit tight, framed by its columns in formal misery. Damp seeps into my legs. Outside the semicircle of our shelter the rain rebounds a foot high above the paving.

After a time, a decent interval as judged by a layman for the cutting and sewing up of the head, we return to the hospital. My scarf has stopped working and I am shaking hard. I leave Vivien on the stairs and as I walk to the door of the Recovery Room I hear a voice. Tom: a man chatting, not even with difficulty but just as exact, as excited as ever, his voice boomy and familiar, and this is a moment like no other. What is it like? Like more than the sum of all the things I have ever anticipated. More. My treat. My gift. Whatever else happens, there will have been this.

The swing door bursts out like a big hello and Mr K, the surgeon, is before me. His eyes fire up to see me and as we conference in the doorway he holds the door ajar with his foot. Water drips from my hair on to my face, from my coat on to the floor and pools around my boots. Mr K is very happy with it. Tom is very happy with it. I am very happy with it.

1.9

Twenty-two thick staples of metal run from below the jaw-line up into the shaved area behind the ear on the left side. From the front you notice nothing, but from the side a blooded silverine line fringed with scabs marks out a wound measuring 12 cm. One week after the operation it has healed well, with no trouble. We have been called back to the hospital to take the metal out and to hear the result of the biopsy. The biopsy is the moment we must submit to, I know that. The result will take us forward in whatever way we go forward but just now the situation with the staples is preoccupying me. The staples are getting in the way. We lean against each other on a pair of green chairs by the entrance to the ward and wait.

There is a machine to do this unpicking and it's a simple tool from a kit a carpet-layer would use. From where we sit, crossways to the bed bays, we can see that there are only two nurses on duty, the German nurse and the one called Donna. Donna has been at various times the nurse assigned to Tom and the relationship has not been good. She is easily embarrassed, whether by him or by every patient she sees, there is no way of telling. It seems unfortunate, cruel somehow on her that she has elected to be a nurse. Her character might come over better as something else, although I'm not sure where her talents lie. She is readily flustered. Items get dropped: urine, blood samples, swabs.

Donna is self-conscious about her body in motion as if aware that she does not do the work well. To cover for this she moves slightly too fast, ever exiting the latest incident. She has been known to pretend not to hear. Her hair is distressed and blonde and fixed up at the back with a stabbed mass of Kirby grips. If she could see herself from behind she would not wear her hair like this.

The choice today is between Donna and the German nurse and whoever is free first will be assigned to Tom. Having watched Donna at work, the idea of her unregulated hands on the hardware to unpin his head makes me hot and weak. I want to cry. I have to stop her.

Charlie the charge nurse comes in. We saw him once in civvies in the lobby, dressed in battered shades of brown and grey and carrying a plastic bag. He looked like a man in a pub. His face is deeply lined, a current or ex-smoker, and in a bar you would not notice him at all. But on the ward he is the only one worth watching. He is the top steward on the cruise ship and he carries his authority carefully and ever so gently separate from himself, as you would a bowl of water. Casual efficiency is ingrained in his manner. He does not hurry but the ward is his domain and he notices everything in it.

He is busy. I have to be quick, seize the moment and step in. *Tom's stitches*, I say to him, *are they going to be done soon*? *When one of the nurses is ready, yes*. No way to finesse this. He must know what she is like. *Can I just ask that it is not Donna*? He has grey eyes the colour of Herdwick wool and he turns them on me. *Yes*.

Charlie is as good as his word. The German nurse takes out the staples very deftly, starting from the bottom, one by one. The bloodied metal brackets clang on to her tray. They look like insects, stuck with matter and bits of hair. In Africa, army ants are sometimes used to do the job of sutures. Here they are simple metal staples. It is no trouble. We wait some more.

We have started to notice a pattern. There are spaces where we are delivered news. They tend to be spaces rather than actual places: generally improvised, porous, makeshift and vulnerable to intrusion. It seems that the delivering of news, however catastrophic, is not regarded as an endpoint in itself but has the status of a transaction done in the open like a piece of knowledge passed from hand to hand on the way to or from somewhere more pressing. Physical interventions – the removal of the staples – are given a site. Yet beyond a single fit, Tom has no symptoms by which we might know he is ill, so knowledge for us is everything. The disease is invisible, and talking about it is the way we feel its charge. Yet we are never presented with sites that might hold a theoretical explosion or contain its profound impact: the dissolution of the floor, folding in of doors and walls, sudden drops in pressure, the creation of a vacuum, the appearance of a void. So all our news, great and terrible, is imparted in liminal spaces. In between. I can name them: the telephone, a pale green transit room opening out on two sides on to adjoining clinics, a swing door, a tiny office crammed with chairs, computers, files and a shredder. This last had a door that could be shut, so it counts at least as a room.

After the removal of the staples and a further half hour waiting, this is where Tom and I; Mr K, the surgeon; and Charlie, the charge nurse meet so that Mr K can give us the biopsy results. The room is so small that once we are seated, in order for anyone to leave we all must rise again. The legs of the four swivel chairs are entangled. No one can exit independently, as the chair-mass blocks the door. The window cannot be opened. A large rubbish bin takes up priority space.

There is no preamble. The biopsy results are as bad as they can be. Grade 4 – *glioblastoma multiforme*. This is the new name we are given. I hear a short suite of words – *aggressive – early – small – encapsulated*. Even in the delivery of wholly violent news I notice Mr K's voice is emollient and slightly hesitant as if to soften the blow, making me think the news might actually be worse in reality even than this. More words are said but the air in the room has fused with the air inside my body, making it difficult for breath to come or go.

This should not be Mr K's job. All praise to the surgeon. He is the one with the good hand and as the bad messenger he is not in his element. His manner and words are functional and in no way sweet as the high art of his knife. We who are good at words would be better than him at this but in this foursome we are suddenly wrong-footed. Something new and strange has happened. We are the victims. I don't know yet what this means but the ground we stand on has gone.

I have to get out in order to think. The news is the whole matter of the meeting so once it is delivered there is little else to say. We rise as a quartet and for a moment the four of us are locked together in an awkward folk dance of non-specific crossing and shaking of hands, symbolic bows of the head, murmurs of thanks and goodwill. What has just happened? We leave.

By heart I know that our route entails a series of right angles, starting with a turn left out of the little room. Thereafter we turn right, out of the ward, out of the hospital, out of the square, out. We walk side-by-side, mute and fused by heat and common danger. My eyes are filmed with fluid that doesn't fall but hangs as a vertical screen. Through it I see the streets are very crowded but I don't notice anything again until we get to the river.

1.10

9 October 2008

Dear Friends

The struggle continues. The biopsy showed that Tom's tumour was malignant. The surgery went very well but he will need a course of radiotherapy, beginning quite soon, and going on for six weeks (that is, going into St Thomas's each day, for a short blast, for five days each week). Tom is otherwise making a good recovery from the operation. He looks and feels well.

The next couple of months of treatment are going to be pretty difficult. So we say again, it's important to us at this time that our friends stay in touch. Please do continue to write, phone, text, email, visit us, and so on.

With love

In September, though deaf to all but our own noise, I pick up the sound of the outside world collapsing. The value of money being wiped off the international markets makes no noise in itself. Loss has local impact. But to the accompaniment of smashing glass and metal, chairs hitting pavements from the fifteenth floor and the collective hum of all the air-cons in America, the big ones go down: Lehman Brothers, AIG, Merrill Lynch, Washington Mutual. Conversely the media goes up like a great big helium balloon. They are making up the deficit in talk. What could be more thrilling than the collapse of the financial systems of the West?

In Clapham after dropping Ev off with a friend I stand on the pavement and stare at a cash machine as if it is a threat. I am there so long someone asks me if I am planning to use it and if not, would I mind moving. My head feels fuzzy and ever so heavy. I would like to rest it on the pavement. I know that our problems are insoluble with money but I wonder if I should be clearing out my bank account.

I leave my pounds where they are. A dream like a brackish stream is going by. I had assumed, like many of my kind, that we would live happily forever. Our future was moored together. We weren't going to divorce, that was clear, and we weren't going to die until we did, in the far distance: old, not without pain but not until a time that made sense, discreetly one before the other or the other way round, leaving a gap, in which whosoever it was who was still living could wonder, drift, mourn, prepare and cease in their turn.

1.11

So what did you do when death came to your house?

We continued in the same way as before.

What is that, a failure of the imagination? Are you in denial?

This is not wholly true; we continue in the same way as before but in parenthesis. My thinking has switched its grammar. The present-continuous is its single operational tense. Uncertainty is our present and our future. Unlike an abstract or esoteric linguistic problem to be puzzled over, this has the force of a wholesale conversion experience. *You are alive, this is your life* becomes *You are alive, this is your life*. Once the nature of the threat is known the defences are brought out at high speed and within multiples of days they are fully rolled out. As well as the surgeon, Mr K, we are assigned an oncologist, Dr B. We are booked to see the neurologist, Dr H. We meet the chemo nurses and Tom is fitted for a radiotherapy mask. We wait for the regime to begin.

But the surface of us appears to be very much the same and this is an early stage intimation of a radical marvel – the flicker between the steadiness of the quotidian and the crash-consciousness of its ending.

To call it even a flicker is an overstatement. The difference between the two states is imperceptible and total. One mindset cannot be attentive to both in the same moment, yet it must. We are in mortal danger and we fall about laughing at what Ev comes up with. We are forever dropping our guard and picking it up. Dropping and picking up are indivisible. They are the same act. The two states are so fused that the switch is not apparent.

Everything living bears the fact of its own dissolution. This is a given. But for us it has become tangible. The universe as experienced is not universal. The universe as experienced is personal. It turns its face towards the individual. It presents an individual form. This individual form is ours. All that adheres will be lost.

Yet there are social and domestic pleasures. And they continue. Decisions that needed to be made two months ago still need making. *What shall we eat? Where shall we go this evening?* I paint our bedroom, not a pressing decision, but what colour should it be? The job has a clear outline, a beginning and end. It is an act of defiance. I crouch on the floor to paint the skirting and hide my face in cornice and cupboard. Low at the carpet where no one will ever look is a long clean edge of white paint at the join of skirting and wall. The line does not waver. I cut corners but I am experienced and I have a good straight hand. The colour of the wall ends up green or perhaps blue, both shades notoriously difficult to assign but the one I choose is deep and saturated. It will soak up all the sunsets that reach us and retain them hard against the retina like a battery.

There was always so much to be done. And now there is so

much more. As Ev gets older the generalia around him multiplies: baby stuff, friends, park, all kinds of play. Tom coming home from hospital brings oxygen back to the house and Ev is invigorated. We see a lot of friends. They all want to come round to verify his continuing existence. Salute the brain. They are reassured. He is the He of He. I welcome them but when they come it's true I remain in tension until they go. I am without conversation and without insight. I have occasional flashes of wit but free-floating, not tied to anything and my words come out impetuous and sudden, like a small child's vomit.

Tom is mending beautifully from the intrusion into his head and we have a string of gorgeous days. Then, one morning ten days in, he has a violent fit. Somehow, though it seems obvious in retrospect, we were not warned that this might happen. It is more disastrous for me than for him. I get to see it. Though it brings an immediate backwash of physical and mental exhaustion, he recovers himself. I do not. I learn something. Here, we commence. We stand at the beginning.

Within the shortest span he starts work again. He picks up his regular writing sooner than anyone can believe. He wants to test his brain, to verify and see what it can do. Every week he writes his pieces for the paper and the work is as it was, complex, active, steady as ever. The words are there for him to find. He can organise the way they flow and the language, its style and rhythm, is his. The text is the proof. He writes slower but with great drive and excitement. He was always very good at this. Under pressure he is getting better.

I am not so mentally well constructed. I am an artist, but making or thinking about making are suddenly out of reach as if they have been confiscated and put away. I do not go to the studio. I no longer understand what the studio is for. What would it be like to be able to think properly? What would it be like to have a thought and set another against it, to make a comparison, formulate an idea? I can't do this. My thoughts, such as they are, run ahead and back like a dog on a tether, covering always the same ground and beating it down to a dry and useless hardness.

I cannot imagine Tom not being with us. I try to imagine futures but can feel my imagination slipping even as I summon them. My mouth is dry. There is no grip. This is my brain in rehearsal and I don't like it. It's a rough, mean-formed thing, like a maltreated animal gnawing and worrying at its new constraints. What I do not imagine is that this is not happening. I am pragmatic. That would be a waste of time.

Tom wants to be treated as an organism. Why not? He's against capitulation in the face of illness, against its distorting power. He will continue as before and fashion it in his image. He is pro-sugar and pro-coffee. Pro-delicious. He is pro his life and the living of it the way he wants to. This is what it means to be an adult. When you have been doing it every day for many years you get used to it. Making decisions. Forming habits. That's what we do.

One of the ways in which ideology manifests is in stroppiness. A refusal to bend in the face of a force outside oneself that seems to be winning. What is the better path: to continue to do things on your own terms, to insist on the primacy and habits of the self, or to adapt? Adaptation leads directly by chute into puzzling terrain. Adapt where? Adapt what? You might conceive of taking decisions as a different person, but what person? Strategies, diets, belief-systems, books, thought-programmes, fads and whole environments exist devoted to change and the 'journey'. It is a self-generated circuit of hell. The Internet is raucous and shouty on all sides about health and its opposite number: pros, cons, pro-cons, pre-cons, dangerous cons, attitudes you never even thought to hold before about subjects you didn't care about till now. We are bored and instantly sceptical but that's our style. We don't think much of choice as it is currently configured. The oncologist, Dr B, is our newest and most clued-up informant and she is careful. She makes precise verbal murmurings only in favour of the evidence-based value of Vitamin C. The NHS recommends a balanced diet. This advice hasn't moved since 1945, so sound is it. Eat well, all things in moderation. OK. Clear enough. So we eat well and we shade towards generous in the moderation. A large tub of high-strength vitamins finds it way on to our shelf.

Pills are new. In the bathroom cabinet we have ibuprofen, ancient paracetamol and tickly-cough mixture for a child. Eye drops from years ago. Indigestion tablets. Calpol. Many things are out of date. We have never had need of drugs. Now we have the steroid dexamethasone, the anti-convulsant Epilim and the chemo drug temozolomide. All are taken at home. The drugs are of such great urgency and moment they capsize us. We do not know how to treat high-octane medicine and give it such symbolic reverence that on the first day we fluff it and the dose spills on the floor. The floor is Ev's domain. He crawls over it, eats toast crumbs from it and picks up dust, rolling it thoughtfully into balls between finger and thumb. My head throbs and my eyes film over as I watch the pills scatter. *We are all going to die.* I am black with anger. We scrabble to find them, count them back in. I think we have them. Minutes later, something digs into my foot through my sock. It is a small white bead of dexamethasone.

And did you rise to what the occasion demanded?

I rose so high, I left my body.

We discover, or rather I do, that you cannot hold a state of fear for an extended time. Fear is a peak, not a plateau. Shock is a drug and at first it feels pure and elevated, yes. The unreal keeps all exalted. Nothing else matters: we are in a state of grace.

But a house can fall down only once and then the dust settles. A train is about to hit and then it does. A wave comes in and sweeps everything away and dead bodies float around in its wash. If you are still alive at this point, you may well die in the aftermath, indeed this seems likely. But terror is a spike. Something else must follow. Terror is followed by less terror, or perhaps – almost inconceivably – by an even worse shock to come. I don't know what the ebb of fear just below the peak is called. It is not a dilution or a lessening but a complexifying. It bears the realisation of what has just happened plus the understanding of what might follow. It is a solid compound of shock plus duration plus comprehension.

After an explosion, if you are still conscious when a blast has happened, everything for you does not cease. There is a shift, a gap, between the impact and the first grasp of what remains and what remaining might entail. What has happened to your body, to the air, to familiar shapes or smells, noise or lack of noise, not like anything there was before? This intermediate time, this ebb, or whatever it may call itself, has a long, slow tail. It leaves a moraine of unconsolidated residue and debris behind. And the tail might last as long as your body continues. Something has happened. The new situation is embodied and you are its witness. This is what happens to me.

1.12

To combat the evil of radiotherapy we decide that good company and minimal hassle are the things to aim for and avoiding the slog into hospital on public transport each day would be a blessing. The radiotherapy rota means organising the friends who have volunteered to drive or accompany Tom for zapping every weekday from Monday to Friday for six weeks. I take this on. My zone of power is so blasted away that like losing weight, this is an area my anxiety can fix on. I go with Tom to the first session and then only once again much later when he asks me to document the experience on video. We are seeking out areas of this thing for me not to be involved in. It is work Tom has to do and he doesn't mind it, or more striking he makes it work for him. In the singular way he can conceptualise his illness he has found here a mode of address. He finds it a kind of pause, a chance to be perfectly *in place*.

He accepts the clamping of the bespoke mask on to his face for what it is: inwardness under restraint. The ray machine is like something from a submarine, a giant upside-down gun turret attached to the ceiling that articulates elegant revolutions around its target. This is precision mathematics. Angle is all. He describes for me the preliminary rituals, lying down, getting settled, strapping in, the nurses' withdrawal behind a shielding screen and their patter to each other as they check and recheck coordinates. They provide music or he can bring in his own. He brings his own. He is the object, helplessly fixed but in charge of himself. Under the ray he can think about what he is writing that week, about living, about dying, us, anything he likes. I dimly get this. I have modelled for drawing classes and drawn from models many times when I was younger: the depersonalisation of the body, the freedom of the mind, the close attention of the eye, the angle of a line, these all fit together. But I mind this process very much. I don't want to see it or be anywhere near it. It is better that only one of us comes here.

Drawing up the schedule is not so difficult. It is an act of solidarity that one can make and there are many volunteers. All I have to do is determine they know the allotted times and dates and keep them informed of the frequent flips in schedule initiated by the hospital. It is not even the case that I do not have anything else to do. Everything else is mine to do. But the radiotherapy schedule signifies something larger than itself. It is an investment: the establishing of a form of order over disaster. I study it endlessly. It looks like something is being done.

The schedule becomes my secret masterwork, though no one else would know it. I do not actually code it in pens of different colours but mentally I do: reds, greens, mauves, yellows and blues, different colours for days of the week, for people of the day, for when the bloods are taken or when the oncologist must be seen or for how long each session will take. I am willing it to work and the way I know how is to pay childish attention to the detail. I am Secretary and Treasurer of the Radiotherapy Club and I carry out my duties to the letter. I will take seriously each tiny seriousness in the hope that they will add up. Each session will be the best it can be. The schedule will fill out its numbers in columns and rows like a sum moving beautifully week after week towards the correct answer.

1.13

23 December 2008

Dear Friends

Happy Christmas to you.

Tom's first round of treatment finished a week ago, and we have a respite until mid-January. So far he's doing well. Ill effects are few and not too terrible.

Thank you for your thoughts, messages, support and company. We look forward to seeing you in the New Year.

With love

On Hampstead Heath six of us are walking. Ev is manfully on his feet, keeping up. He measures 70 cm high. We have the buggy with us but when he is tired he simply bends his tummy and folds softly on to the winter grass. It is a fierce day, chill, with a bright blue sky.

Nobody talks very much yet this is a kind of celebration. We are three months since the operation. Tom looks radiant. His eyes are brilliant blue and his hair the darkest brown. None of his hair has been lost. It hangs slick over his forehead in a neat curtain, covering the scar on the left side with ease. The rays of radiotherapy are bouncing off him and the schedule is over. His skin always looks fantastic, the skin of a young man. Ev is radiant too. He has good reason to be. We are out with friends in the open. He is the only child in a group of adults and orchestrates our attention. Picking our way through the sharp end-of-year grasses, we gather sticks and leaves to present to him and then chase him round a ring of birches dappled in camouflage of black and white bark and green and yellow leaves. He is an easy catch, stiff with nappy, buttoned up in his blue winter coat. When caught, he folds and squeals like a young pig. His legs kick the air.

On the turn towards Kenwood we walk through the area of birches where dogs and dog-walkers make their meet. A woman with five dogs on radiating leads: brown, grey, black, white, brindled, meets a man with three: black, tan and mouse and another man with two: white and spotted. Dogs and guardians congregate in delight. It is like an open-air revivalists' meeting. They socialise in happy circles. Ten dogs sniff each other's arses in swirling motion. If they could applaud, they would.

I know this bit of ground well. Five summers ago I filmed here over several days researching the terrain. My viewpoints were always particular features lined up through the lens. Mainly I was looking at edges: landscape clusters, paths, trees, mounds, rocks, and how they might be outlined and digitally rendered into vignettes like small solids or floating islands, free of the standard rectangle of the lens. I digitally removed the sky. Left only the land and its adherent trees. I had been thinking of Bewick the engraver and how self-sufficient his illustrations are, each a summons to a place on a white page. In a Bewick vignette, all living takes place within a conscious edge. The shape frames the action. It is not a contingent view. You cannot step out. There is no out. There is no elsewhere, nothing external, no shift of angle to the right or pulling back the shot to reveal the whole. Strange reciprocity: the figure and its scene are birthed together.

I filmed in the circle of trees where we chase Ev. Another clump of oak and lime on the hill, a third view round the turn of the main serpentine path as it slips away. Much of it didn't get used, but there was one path nearby with a precise jaunt and sweep away from the lens that made it in. I haven't been back much since and as I recognise each site my eye returns to those familiar decisions of edge and shape and outline. This is what I was looking at then. Now I am not selecting. I don't have the camera but the limits of my visual field. My family and my friends are in the shot. There is no elsewhere.

Ev sits on Tom's shoulders. He is too tired to walk any more. His mouth is open and he makes a husky singing note in his throat. The pitch does not waver. A tiny cloud of breath hangs in front of the O of his mouth. As Tom starts to jog away along the dirt track the note gets muddled and starts to vibrate and when Ev notices this, a new note of laughter mixes with the sound. Tom jogs faster. The first note cannot hold. It continues but dissolves from song into laughter held at the same pitch. His head falls back, giggling, helpless.

1.14

Sometime towards the end of January Ev is ill and he vomits on the rug. As I can't think what to do with it, I roll it up and throw it down the back steps into the garden. The afternoon passes. He buries his face in the sofa, mooning his white bottom at me. A papery moth flits out of a cushion and I crush it between my fingers. Moths are eating all our wool. The sky outside is metallic and the trees are bare of leaves.

Holed up in close proximity with Ev, his conversation is a surprise as always. Sickness marginally drags his spirits but makes his talk spacier, bouncier. *This is my knee* – he sits on the floor caressing it. He puts the toy ambulance in a jam jar – *Look, I've made a yoghurt*. Then he pushes the ambulance around on the table – *Beep beep – ambulance goes to the hospital for daddy*. Today, being ill, we are idle. The rhetoric on childcare doesn't much do idleness, preferring the term 'work'. Being a mother I am now an expert but I still find that what we do remains slippery and hard to categorise: avoidance, whimsy, indulgence, play. Lying on the sofa and making a long hill for his car with my body, throwing cushions at him, pretending to sleep and having him burrow in beside me then collapsing him by sniffling my nose around in his neck whispering *I smell truffles*. These things are known to be good for children. They are good for me and good for him and if I didn't do them his life and mine would be the poorer. I am no stranger to idleness but I had no idea my life lacked this. What I did before I had him was as variously urgent, vital, exciting, mundane, novel or boring as any life. I never noticed a gap in it for this.

Tom is a little bit in awe of Ev, of his resilience and inventiveness. Ev has the baby fur of self-possession. He goes around the house humming tunes to himself that he doesn't like us to join in on. The fluid natter of his makey-up play-world is a comprehensive universe packed with verbal surprises. He can take himself off to nap in the middle of the day like a cat. He has sentences and phrases that he uses to probe the material around him – *Oh! Hmm, OK, perhaps this, Hmm – what could this do?* He has started nursery. There they call him *The Deep Thinker*. Ev already knows a great deal about himself, his needs, his powers, what makes him happy. He knows us well too, senses prevarication and is surprised by falsity. His face melts to tears at slights. He can spin a situation round from desperate to blithe in a moment. We are both surprised by the fecundity of his naughtiness. He has a brilliant memory for his mayfly past and once you work out what he is talking about, he is invariably right. A child can do this, flaunt itself and its knowledge, continuously brand new, and then newer still. It can chomp through words; making the rapid, raw, connecting work of jumps, jokes, new meanings, confusions, mishearings and rhyming nonsense. Yesterday Ev noticed a bush in the park, neat as a lollipop. *If that tree were choc-o-late I would eat it.*

I've mainly missed what the others talk about: trials, desperation, panic. Not lack of sleep. I didn't miss that. I had it and have it still. My nights are a negative of my days. The lack of sleep I now have is grievous but Ev is not its true cause. But the rest wasn't so all-encompassing. It seemed to last about six beats. Already he is not a baby and his babyhood feels elided, glossed. Maybe all mothers feel this, but it as if I am easily deceived concerning him. My memory is selective.

I forget about the two miscarriages that preceded him. I do not mean to do this. It's not something I am consciously trying to do. It is not a boast. But it shows how strong is Ev's grip. In Glasgow, I decide to look up a friend I haven't seen for years. Vulnerability is making me bolder and more restless. I contact her and seek her out, and Ev and me go on a straggly bus journey from the city centre to the edge. At the designated spot there she is waiting for me, hands in pockets, same as she was. She has two teenage children, thin as zips, and as we settle in with each other over the course of the next hours she tells me of her difficulties getting pregnant. She asks, *How was it for you? Oh, it was OK,* I say, *it kind of happened.* About a week later I recall this conversation suddenly and am astonished. What a lie! Two miscarriages isn't such a carefree path to pregnancy. I was forty-two when I gave birth. It was not seamless. It did not just kind of happen. But while speaking to her I had been looking at Ev and my mind was on him. It is more than forgetting or suppressing. It is the utter refutation of the existence of anything else. He sweeps all before him. All the non-and-never-children are lost in his black shadow, in the gleam of his silver reflection. With him, the present trumps the past, always. This will stand him in good stead.

1.15

Ev passes his sickness on to me. Tom, whose immunity is so compromised, is spared. The day I am well enough to leave the house it snows heavily and lies so thick the city calls a truce. With each hour more of its functions cease. For now the Whites have it. Some quarters struggle on, others lay down their arms and citizens emerge from their homes. Fearful that it will not last, I scramble to get Ev out in the optimal hush.

In countries where it is rare, deep snow is the people's bounty and the park at 3 p.m. is packed with revellers. They all do the same thing, not minding repetition or convention or at all; sliding downhill on trays and Tesco bags, pelting each other and rolling balls of dirty snow taller than themselves to leave them parked at random like abandoned trailers. Tom comes out to meet us, walking carefully with a stick. He loves snow and will not miss it. The light is brilliant and reflects back into our faces. We look well.

We are post-radio, deep in chemo. When Tom is exhausted and the evening collapses for him around seven o'clock, after Ev is put to bed, I think of the hours that lie ahead without his company. At this point if I am in such a mood for it I become angry. Dark begins to settle in at four. I consider the options: 1 stare into space, 2 drink, 3 eat, 4 book, 5 wash clothes, 6 tidy up toys, 7 keep warm, 8 phone someone, 9 we do not have a television so that option is out, 10 is anything which requires special initiative. Quite often 1 has it. The snow has appeased me but my temper circuits around itself at this hour and can catch Ev if he is not asleep in time. It is a tightly wound little lash of foulness that will suddenly show its tip with a near total lack of build-up and even as it hits it is splashed and watered with contrition.

Yet I keep saying to people, *You have got to realise that we are having a very good time*. I am saying this while explaining that Tom has this thing and everything, the whole attendant works, gunning for him. I repeat it many times, especially at the beginning, and though I know it to be true, I can see they don't believe me. I can tell by their eyes, their ever-ready nodding and murmuring. *It's good you are so strong. You've got to be positive*. I give up after a while, but it continues to annoy me and I nag away at trying to find a form of words for having a life consistent with this paradox. I don't succeed. The sentence – *We are happy because we can hold totally opposite positions in equilibrium in our heads at the same time, though you might not realise beforehand that this is possible* – is not one you can use in many conversations.

He is dying. Yet within the context of *us*, this fact can seem irrelevant. I might sometimes say, *So what?* This is not the same as denial. It is simply that our understanding of each other is unchanged and will not change until this is over. It sticks to us like spray on skin. *He loves. He is loved. He has loved. He will be loved.* Being with a long-time love is having the shape and expanded sweep of their person annexed to yours. It is a psychic extension that generates surprising patterns through which things pass unnoticed, move, switch and flood back. It is as near as thinking, as regular as breathing and yet you are not quite aware of its limits. Knowing your own limits, where you yourself begin and end so well as to be dulled by them, its pleasure derives precisely from the ambivalence of not knowing where the edges lie, yet feeling at home.

1.16

It isn't true when I said that I sometimes phone people. I do not. Never. I am even out of that habit. People must phone me. This business of getting on with it is very singular. Talking about what is happening to us opens up great holes and hidden traps. I cannot allow this too often and I must ration the demands that such conversations have on me.

After much mental preparation, *Shall I, Shan't I*, and the taking on and pulling off of clothes as I choose my armour with care, I go out to a gallery for the private view of an exhibition of the artist Liz Arnold. The personality of the paintings hits as soon as you enter the room. It is an interior kind of world. Small canvases in ice-cream colours; strawberry, black, turquoise and lime, sprinkled with silver and gold dust and loaded with neon highlights and wonky patterns. The world depicted is clearly London, peopled by characters much like ourselves, awkward and delicate, prone to embarrassment and easily upset. Except that they are ants, small insects, shy bees or flamboyant creatures with thin legs and wings. The paintings are clever and witty and turbulent, with shades of Alex Katz in the slabby blankness of the painting but with a disco fizz and a gaucheness that slips between the familiar and the very odd indeed.

The place is packed. I never knew her but she was a popular figure, much missed, and the crowd is hugely partisan. They are reconnecting, happy and excited to see her singular universe reframed. The world of people who might know these paintings is a small one. I know many of them and if they know me, then they also know us and will know what is happening to us.

I have made the wrong decision in coming out. A big, avoidable error and now I must manage the consequences. The situation is too fraught. Old friends yes, I can sidle up to them and hug, elide or glide past as I wish, but the others, the acquaintances, the professionals, the half-known, the supposed-to-know, what am I to do with them? What is there to say? I try to focus on the paintings but on entering the room my skull has become illuminated. An internal bulb or light has gone on and I am incandescent and highly spottable. News is news, and the badder the news, the harder it is to avoid. I am no longer myself, solo person, viewer, artist, colleague, friend of somebody else, whatever, but I am that person, the person who is married to the person who ... *Oh there she is, that is her, yes I heard, oh God and yes, they've got a child too.*

I am not long in the gallery before someone makes a beeline for me. I can see her mouth making shapes and framing questions already as she advances through the crowd, the standard ones I know, but ever harder to field. I am struggling even before she reaches me. My illuminated skull flickers in panic. Another one appears from the right with the same aim in mind. They do not know each other, yet they have a common animal zeal: to support me. Am I supposed to introduce them? They want facts: information, details, prognosis; they both have stories of colleagues, friends, people they don't know themselves, who have overcome this or that tumour. Their eyes are wide for the task. It is a double-headed attack and I am trapped in the clash of their antennae. I am at a private view holding a glass of wine in the middle of a crowd of anthropomorphic insect paintings and I am being devoured by deadly human mouthparts. I last as long as I can, but really it is minutes, no time at all, and in between one word and the next my feet lock to the straightest line through the crowd to the door. By instinct and not by sight I get out, drinking great sobs and heaves with tears glassing my face as I run.

With different details, people, places, this scenario happens many times. Sometimes I manage to have more fun before breaking down, sometimes not. At a certain point the only way to guard fully against it is to stay at home or circumscribe ever closer the people I meet. But we keep at it, these ventures: holding on to things, to people, like lamp-posts in fog. It seems we must. We inhabit a physical world where the number of places to go and people to encounter is vast but finite. This is held to be a good thing. Imagine its opposite. The same spaces and people that held us before must hold us now.

If we were spirits we would use crisis as an opportunity to flit, change shape, become airborne or take to the trees. We might change from water to wood, or wood to wind. Embodiment feels like a dull strain, an afterthought. It gives me a headache. Socially, I am near unobtainable. Tom does much better, and Ev, our ambassador, the best. As physical creatures our movements remain linear, horizontal and heavily patterned to fit our environment. It is inescapable. We accept an invitation, leave the house, walk to the station, down the escalator, take the Tube, up the stairs and go out into the world as guests.

It doesn't happen this way to Tom. He is special. I am in sum a reporter to events. The worst is not happening actually to me but conversely, as we both acknowledge, that puts me further out in danger. I have the job of wholly partial observer. I am a commentator. I am therefore unarmed. He has the sword and mighty shield, the gravitas of the very seriously ill.

1.17

In mourning, wrecked before the fact, I try counselling. It's been nine months since this thing started. I am against going forward as I don't want the thing that is going to happen to happen. The future is not mine, nor is it Ev's. The future is against us.

Round One of counselling is on the NHS. The hospital is a complex growth by the side of the Thames. It is architecture by accretion. Any planning was contingent on decisions made before and like a hand-drawn line which tries to echo another hand-drawn line and then another, it quickly deviates and no longer looks anything like its line of origin. I am directed to a temporary building on the roof of an annexe to the main body. This is the counselling department. From the ground it looks like a box a child might stick on top of a fort made of other boxes: a provisional outpost that was built for expediency and got stuck. Its route is signposted along a series of increasingly dismal corridors. The journey takes many convoluted minutes and signals long before you arrive the low cultural status within the hospital of the talking art as a mode of healing. The walk, and the experience of the waiting room when you get there, are so crushing it is worth not going so as not to experience either of them. The neutral decor is an assault. I last two sessions.

I wish that someone, anyone – any of these people who are paid to do this – would actually just tell me what to do. *Bring what you will to the session,* says the therapist. She settles back in her chair and eyes me with sympathy. Her eyes are filmy. I can see myself and the windows of the room reflected in their whites. She is passive. I have not yet opened my mouth and I am defeated.

I have many friends skilled in sympathy. Strategy is what I need. I need tactics: a manager, coach, a trainer who knows about the death stuff. After all, dying is not unknown. It is astonishingly common for all that we regard it and there are a multitude of facts which can be addressed: about the understanding of young children, about the deep fatigue generated by stress, about what illness does to concentration, about financial support, about anger, the family, stasis, identity, love, society and all the skeins involved in the ravelling out of the whole.

I have my topics on a piece of paper. They are:

1. The question of grief in advance
2. Being stuck in the present
3. The nature of uncertainty
4. Other people

Round Two occurs some months later. A friend recommends a small agency specialising in cancer that works with patients and family. The decor of the place is progressive: solid, warm, dark colours in heavy peppermint greens and aqua blues. It is a tiny dedicated outfit where a clutch of trained counsellors work for not much money and have to spend a large portion of their time fund-raising instead of talking to clients. The sessions are affordable as they are heavily subsidised.

My topics are still the same, but this time the approach is pragmatic and strategic. Here is a case. A catastrophe. An emergency. It is all hands on deck. Most of the time in the sessions I am crying. But in the gaps, when I stop, I begin to speak. So a fragment can be brought to light and we both try to look at it sideways so that incrementally, week by week, a picture of what it looks like may form. I have never cried like this. The fatigue of it is seismic. This is crying as main violence to the self. Its aftermath is like the aftermath of assault: shock, exhaustion, confusion, with the sessions resonating in my head like tinnitus that ebbs slowly over days.

The shock feels greater because the tears are my first intimation of scale. I am nearing the iceberg. My tears are sonar. They release on impact a faint understanding of what lies beneath: a vast solid, the floating mass of ice that is still to come. These are early days.

Acclimatisation is a curse and a blessing and it becomes clear that from my position at the heart of the gathering chaos I can scarcely see anything at all. I am caught between adrenalin and its back-drag, inertia. Tom is months into chemo. He sleeps as a man drugged, but when awake he works and his work goes slower but with great clarity. Not less than normal. Not more than normal. The same. Exhaustion blankets the house. We are always between scans, the one past and the one to come. We live out each three-month instalment while tiny fits explode on us like bombs lobbed from outside. Ev becomes bolder and wilder.

The sessions give me a weekly platform from which to look at the rushes of my life as I live it. God what a madhouse! It is astonishing, intolerable. Save everyone! It must be stopped.

1.18

The oncologist, Dr B, is always of interest. It takes me a session or two to get used to her. At first I think her eyes have too much potential to show alarm but this is before I understand what alarm there is. We are glad it is Dr B. That she is the one if one needs to be had. She is a fait accompli: here is the cancer and here the cancer doctor. It turns out by chance that Tom knows her through a loose connection of friends and flat-shares a decade past. She has spent that decade getting very good at her job as he has spent his, so it seems not incongruous that they should meet again in this setting. It is somehow appropriate. Connection is a good thing.

At first it disconcerts the bureaucracy. *Would you rather have someone else*? they ask, as if the relationship between patient and clinician should properly be sealed, vacuum-tight in the world of the unwell with no leakage. We are crossing the Styx. Cancer exists everywhere embodied in major and minor forms yet this sanctity is strongly held. We find it so hard to address it that we bequeath the disease great privacy and shade. It is its own shroud. *No*, Tom says, and he is right. That he already knows Dr B allows him immediate access and means that there are sometimes other things to talk about apart from the tumour and its workings. After all, there are always other things to talk about.

In reality between dawn and dusk we might not talk about it much at all though we hold it in our minds. Tom says he does all the time, though you would never know it. For me it sits as if on the curve of a graph from near to far that can slip for short periods over the horizon, usually when I am thinking about Ev. The relationship with the oncologist sets up something like a good mood or a background pattern to an appreciation that kicks in very easily. She makes herself exceptionally open to us. Whether this is true for all the others we never find out, but we have her mobile number and on that bright morning ten days after surgery when I found Tom speechless and flailing she answered it directly. Dr B responds promptly to emails and our dialogue with her is unlike any other we have. Something different from a friendship, it is sudden, expedient, contingent yet wholly actual. This is no small comfort.

In the affectless spaces of the hospital basement where Cancer and Chemo live, her fitted dresses and suits suggest flamboyance under restraint and she is a sight I look out for. She comes into view like a yacht. I always notice what she is wearing and am cheered by it. She likes a flared skirt with a strict belt and an outfit with an asymmetric cut. Minus the twenty-first-century tailoring, it's the New Look. She takes a heel and there is always a point in these sessions to stare at the floor so I look at her shoes. They are dramatic.

The other basement workers wear blue belted dresses or wide, white tunics and trousers. On their feet they all have Crocs. Their bodies could be happily drawn and coloured-in with crayon going well over the outline while hers always seems delineated and freshly scored in sharp pencil. She works unfathomable hours and sometimes phones late at night. From the background noise, she calls from everywhere: taxis, stairwells, the office, the street, stations, on the way to other meetings.

Dr B is our teller of news, good and mainly bad, and she has charge of the rich implications that can be given over in the voice and analysed into the nuances, said and unsaid, that continue after the voice stops. Dr B can picture in her head the likely arc of the disease and has seen it plotted live many times against a timeline. A blizzard of lines echoing each other at the start, some surprising misfires, shortfalls, divergences and then long lazy reaches of line continuing as the others fall away. It is a contingent arc. She knows not to describe everything at once.

In sessions our talk is compressed. She works against the clock and there are many patients to be seen, though this is a pressure we feel lightly: again, a mark of her efficacy. This is serious and you have to do it right. Yet we can make her laugh, especially Tom. As a third party I see that doctor and patient are on some level amazed at each other. She at his mode of being with disease, at the integrity of his identity as it progresses, and he at her vigilance against it. In clinic, his amazement can extend again, vivid as it ever first was, simply to his situation as he narrates it. He is telling her each fresh adventure he has and there is pleasure in this too for both of them. Her eyes widen with laughter as she looks at us and narrow again as she leans to consult her notes.

1.19

I dream of a response. It troubles me like a rash, like a whole-body itch that needs to be relieved. A public response is what I'm after. Here is my idea so you can see how inadequate it is. I will make a costume to be worn every day as long as we both last. Wearing it, I will be identified with him and by association with his illness. I am not ill. I am not mad. I do not have Münchausen's. I am a witness. And what may a witness do?

For its design I look to the vanguardists of the West and further East, the former GDR or Bauhaus: Rodchenko, Malevich, Schlemmer. We go to an exhibition of the Dutchman Van Doesburg and admire his ingenuity getting stuck into everything: tiling, trousers, streamlined stools and schools in primary colours, social housing, all practical and optimistic in the Dutch way. I lived for four years in Amsterdam. Better design makes better public life, they say. Better public life makes better life. I imagine a thick felt suit in black and camel or an aubergine and lime livery with hints of London transport. This preoccupation lasts many weeks and it is born of anger. I won't have a discreet coloured ribbon or a cool, confident young person's T-shirt. I am looking to construct an irrefutable suit, an awkward carapace that is something like armour. I feel warped, unrecognisable. So why is this not visible? My idea doesn't fit into existing modes of public consciousness-raising. It would mark me out as trouble, a tumour bag lady. Tom understands, though he finds such an idea ridiculous. It is ridiculous. Though the problem lies in cells, truly disempowerment is continuous with the problem.

A dad who has learned of our situation comes up to me in the playground. I loathe the playground as much as Ev loves it. It is ripe for Council uplift: exposed tarmac, peeling paint and knackered railings, no soft landings. The place is hard and gives no solace. This is a nice dad. He offers to help in any way he can and shaking his head tells me that knowing of our trouble has put his rows with his wife about money into perspective.

Hunched on the bouncy horse, I watch Ev in the sandpit trade diggers like a merchant making a profit. Folded in this position I am stuck, my hips are trapped and my legs curled under me. I am an allegorical figure turned in on herself, an emblem, a symbol for others. Nicolas de Larmessin, the French engraver, made a series of prints of tradesmen, grotesquely fleshed with the apparatus of their trade: butcher, hatter, knife-and-scissor-sharpener, all solid and stiff as sandwich boards. A satire on *The Dance of Death*, he called it *The Dance of Work*. My trade would be Bad-luck-measurer. I could wear the fussy brocade of Victim, the slashed coat of Not-so-fortunate, the rough dress of Never-so-bad-as-that. Then in the street and in the playground I would be taken as a rule, a living testament to mortality and to the acquisition of perspective. People say that children put everything into perspective and then they say that again about the dying. What do they say the rest of the time? Why, they don't care about perspective at all.

But even as I fret, I know it will go nowhere. It is clear that my costume would only stand as a gesture of the most superficial kind. I might twist it one way or another, yet the sub-text, rather than being an act of solidarity, is simply its opposite. The garment could only draw the eye from him to me, from his cause to mine, for I would be sure not to devise a dress that made me look anything other than striking, or anything other than mad – and therefore equally striking – worthy of pity and attention. Me. Me. Me too. That's what the costume would say. It doesn't escape my notice either that the regular channels for public response or consciousness-raising in our situation, running marathons or fundraising for community initiatives, don't cross my mind. Medicine is providing the vanguardism and the cutting-edge ideas. Dressing up falls woefully behind the curve. The wind has gone out of me. Mortality is making me conventional. The costume is not made.

1.20

6 June 2009

Dear Friends

It's been a while since we sent one of these out, not since December. The months seem to have passed quickly. Tom is about to have his last week of chemo, which will mark the end of this round of treatment. After that, there will be a scan. After that, we're not sure.

So far he continues to feel very well. He is doing his work as normal. But this has now been going on for a long time and it has affected us differently. It's been a lot of strain for Marion, less so in some ways for Tom, and none at all apparently for Ev, who continues to flourish.Thank you again for your thoughts, messages, support and company. We look forward to hearing from you.

With love

Ours is a slow house. Nothing much is visible from the outside. The curtains are drawn. Treatment is the alternative calendar of our days. Like a corrupted menstrual cycle, Tom has been on chemo drugs taken at home for five days, followed by a slow disengagement over twenty-eight. He takes it well. So far ill effects are few. The desire for sleep and the difficulty of getting it is our main trial. In the earliest hours of a morning as Ev comes in and grinds his skull yet again into mine, I push him roughly from the bed. *Just Go Away*, I shout.

I am still breastfeeding. Ev grows in our sight. Then one evening he has a drink, just a small suckle, when his attention is distracted by something else: a curl of silver paper, a toy car, a noise on the stairs. After that, nothing. Finished. The child is distracted forever.

Tom goes into hospital to pick up his pills, get his blood checked and see Dr B. Otherwise we operate like norms. Tom works. I work such as I can. We live socially. We go to the cinema, to the galleries and out into the city but our movements are careful and measured. We are watchful.

These are our days. Our nights are another matter. For Tom, lying down is painful and sleep precipitates waking. Insomnia rules the house. His body is uncoordinated and when he turns he can do it only by throwing himself repeatedly over and over in increments, like a man in a sack. The bed bangs and shakes. I am awake. I seem to be always awake though this cannot be true or I would be dead. We are like exhausted mammals, finned creatures, beached. We have tried sleeping separately. That didn't work and anyway we want to be together. We can be more inventive than that.

Before illness, me being the worst nurse was an open joke. This has not changed. I find it hard. For six months Tom has been on steroids. Their purpose is anti-inflammatory, reducing the swelling in the brain around the tumour. His dose is low at the moment, 1mg per day, but steroids are a notoriously short-term line of defence. Over time they turn on the body and wear it down, weakening the muscles. When you bring the dose down, as he is doing now, it is debilitating. The muscles have to be built up again.

For weeks movement is a struggle. The aches are highly mobile and come to rest in the oddest places, the cusps or outside edges of his hands or the backs of calves. Pain flicks too round the shoulders, thighs, knees, so fitful that it is impossible to plot a defensive strategy. He is useless at exercise and in these extreme conditions continues to be so.

Another's constant complaints are boring, that is known. Also this moaning is in a secondary league. He is not saying *I am in pain from the tumour,* which I would be a monster of cruelty not to react to, but *I am in pain everywhere all the time for cumulative reasons that are not immediately life-threatening.* This is so vague, and so much the bedrock of our situation, that I can only be fitfully empathetic. So I am not empathetic enough. I am too tired, too busy. Pulling his weight is not in question. Not literally. Not figuratively. Nights are endurance courses over the distance.

But nothing is unbearable. We find that everything can be accommodated and everything can be tried at least once. Whole sleep-theories are extrapolated out of a single precious night of half-decent rest. *Why did that work? Maybe we should try this? Was that a little better?* Time is so tricksy I cannot track it. Two nights is eternity. We endure continuously everything all at the same time. The good happens in the maw of the bad and the bad in the teeth of the good. I am a saint, I tell you, in what is expected of me here. It is a monstrous evil this sainthood. A deformity. Worn like a caul. We have gone into Bible time. It is medieval. It is more primitive than you can imagine.

1.21

On Brockwell Park we stand with our backs to the slope. Mornings when we open the curtains, each time the sky is the same colour. I don't know what to do about this. It is in some way a direct offence against us but there it is. Same blue. It forces us to go with it, to set in motion the things a sunny day demands. With a child you fall into patterns of activity so days end up both different and the same, same setting, subtly different child, acquisitiveness enlarging his arena each day. It is accretion by pushing: relentless, local and undistinguished.

It is easiest to stay close near Tom and near home, so often that means the park. Ours sits on a hill from where you can see a tranche of London realigned and even though I know the view so well, it remains slightly mysterious. The major landmarks in parallax interrupt the skyline in a way that isn't quite right, and look slightly daft in contrast with the more conventional view – or perhaps the conventional view is simply from the north. Buildings miles away bank up and dwarf each other on the same sightline. Shard, Gherkin, Wharf, Eye. It is a collage.

The park serves many functions. For Ev it is an entrée to dogs and dirt and strangers and the act of running away. For Tom it is his constitutional as he weans himself off chemo. The gentle walk up the hill along and down helps open out the muscles of his thighs, soften his legs and invigorate his head. The very known-ness of the place means he can sleepwalk. We always came here. Now it is imperative. Whenever Tom suggests a walk I never turn it down.

We arrive in the park in all combinations. Tom alone with a book, us three in a loose unit, Tom and a friend, me and he marching in close step, a whole troupe of us messing about on the slopes. Ev has a weekly appointment with a dog to gouge leaves from drains and throw sticks. One permutation has ended though. Ev and Tom don't come here together. The risk of a fit while Tom is alone with Ev unmarked in the wide space is more than we can bear. We did it for a while, and now we don't. This is a secondary and unforeseen by-product of illness and its impact blankets an expanse of our activity.

We come here in all weathers but there is only one weather currently on offer and the blue becomes more exacting as the days go by. Crossed vapour trails mark out the spot above our heads. *Here they are! Here!* Often we bring lunch or supper with us: dahl, rice, chicken green masala with poppadoms bigger than our heads. Ev will tear through these by himself. We eat falafel with hummus and pita or we forget about food and bring a bottle of Prosecco, setting the bottle to fire askew into space between us, its base manipulated neatly into the dirt.

These days I am always looking for a place on which to rest my eyes, for some sight that might be neutral and tolerable and will not hurt me. If I could shut my eyes for a month, I would. But because I know this park so well and know it all so well in the company of Tom, the sight of it now pains me very much. Here is hard evidence for the external world as construct. In all our excursions is the imprint of past excursions. You wouldn't even call them walks: arrivings and standings-still, alternated with movement, roundels and circuits. To be aimless in the company of another is a fine aim. This is one of the bits of ground on which we have tested each other's measure over a long time. This is where our thoughts have been salted with new thoughts. But it means that every bit of this municipal land incorporates the future. To visit *my* park, the park of habit and memory, is to glimpse a projection of the time when we will no longer come here together. It is a whitish projection, not clear, something like a thin line thrown blindly ahead, a trajectory of spit, a nebulous strand without substance. Future walks. Future halts. Stops.

Unlike falling in love, there will be no period of grace in which to work out how to be apart. It will just happen. I *will* experience this place in the future without him by my side. So what I see on the ground here is this. The path curving upward to the house with the land falling away right and left on either side. The runnel of grass that intersects the imprint of the cricket nets. The usual bench we gravitate towards. The pointed spire from Samuel Palmer that spikes the horizon in the direction we never take. And this is what I see when I look closer: Tom's eyes shaded under his hat. Ev's jacket dropped on the path. The pushchair with a collection of sticks and leaves mounting on its hood. And closer still: my hand in his, Ev's hand in his, their silhouettes as they move ahead of me big and small against the sun.

Ev likes to sit within sight of the miniature railway that is staffed at weekends in summer by men who bring the trains in from the suburbs on the roof-racks of their cars. Through the week, children shuttle along the vacant line and the little boys are programmed to follow it from end to end. They get as much neurotic pleasure from this as they do from riding the train. Up until the age of about five their feet are the wrong gauge. They pitch and wobble over the sleepers, falling off and righting themselves. Touching the buffers makes Ev happy. In reverse, he will jump categories with impunity and make a noise like a lorry in retreat.

In these weeks of local sun everlasting and blasting, my understanding of the dialectic of terminal illness at its most intricate is growing to make a bank of observations and a bank of hurt exactly corresponding. *What You Love You Will Lose*. All these records are thrown together, not filed, but interleaved hastily like cards with no chronology, and the entries in this archive are mounting up now into the thousands. I do not know who will ever look at this archive. I do not know where its limits will be. From the top of the park, backs to the slope, above our heads, the sky ascends as immaculate as the skies in *Les Très Riches Heures,* their colours matched directly to the Virgin's cloak.

We are creatures of context. We can only see as far as we can see. I can only think in the way that I can think. The sky only appears blue. Beyond our view we know that it will edge from blue to dark, from dark to black, away from the atmosphere and hard pull of the earth. There is something here I did not know before. I thought that there were limits to the absorption of pain. I thought that it was finite. I thought that it would stop.

1.22

17 July 2009

Dear Friends

Tom had a scan last week. Yesterday we were given the results. They were described as 'very good news'. Since the last scan in January the affected area of his brain has shrunk, and there are currently no signs of bad activity there.

This is obviously encouraging, not least because we weren't expecting anything so definite. But the situation is ongoing and there will be another scan in three months' time.

Thanks again for your thoughts, messages, support and company. We look forward to hearing from you.

With love

The summer is taking shape and it is the shape of France. This is unusual. I have never been on a French holiday in the way the English do. This summer we go there twice. Tom is well enough that it feels beneficial for the three of us in a nineteenth-century way to move out of our sphere and take the air in another. We move from bad spores toward good, from the miasma into the brisk air. The outcome of the latest scan translates into speech as *Very Good*. *Good* and *Bad* are the sum total of the standard descriptors up till now. It is either one or the other and the language is never tarted up, so *Very Good* is an outcome we must celebrate. *Very Good* gives us a rocket of energy like a burst of ticker tape, a firework display, a rain of glitter from heaven. An unreadable scan counts as a nothing, a nil or the equivalent of not having had an MRI at all. No change of course comes into the category *Good*. *Very Good* means we go on holiday. A holiday from watchfulness is all I seek.

As we don't plan holidays, often they don't turn up. Through my twenties I played in a band and we toured a great deal in Europe and America. This has made me insensitive to tourism. Travel was a by-product of work. We were always going to places to meet people who wanted us to come in order to hear and see the things we did. To go to a place without being invited still seems genuinely foreign, like pretending you lived temporarily somewhere else. Why would you do that? Tom never cared much about travel. What he needs is in his head and hands, and in us.

July: We are in a wooden house in Brittany. It faces the beach. Three generations ago it was hard against the sand. Then a road was built to join the scattered houses to the village. The road was later widened as more visitors came, then parking bays were introduced and now a further barrier of angled parking fringes the view with a buffer of silver and black estates. Bull bars against the ocean. As the cars get higher and heavier: vans, trailers, 4 x 4s, sailing kit, the view becomes ever more impeded until evening falls, when suddenly they all depart again, leaving us to sit on the step in the hazy late sun.

Nights are sweet and blue, with the lights ribboning into the distance as we walk along the promenade. The town has a neat modern centre and smells of burnt sugar, nougat and toffee. Our friends, whose extended family owns the house, have been coming here for steadfast local pleasures for years: eating and swimming, low-level reading and talking. It is delicious to be a guest in someone else's life. Our family has been taken up temporarily into theirs with low expectations of us and we may safely drift even below them. Tom sleeps chemo-sodden sleeps.

Very early, before the cars arrive to take their slots, Ev and I fall out on to the beach for our private sessions between six, when he wakes, and nine, when the household does. I take a cup of coffee with me and caffeine resonates like a gong in my head in time with the light bouncing off the sea. My eyes are slits. The air sparkles. The beach is glitter and pearl. Most mornings we meet two people, the man who does Tai Chi and outlines the yin-yang slowly in the sand with a stick, and the big wet woman who swims with her big wet dog. For the rest, the beach is empty. Ev and I are incandescent. We chase each other across yellowness. He is golden as he watches blood-warm water trickling on to his toes, in and out, in and out. He says nothing but learns by feel about tides and pull, gravity, planets and moons.

Wood ingrained with salt and sand is the matter of the house. Summer dries it, winter wets it, expansion and shrinkage go in yearly cycles and whole feet and inches might be added to its size over a season. The floors gape with gigantic knot holes. Panelling, stairs, the arms of chairs and ancient bookcases, all are rubbed and handled to a sensual smoothness. Ev plays with wooden bricks from thirty years ago. Their paint is worn away to rare un-nameable hues. Every colour in the house has muted and his plastic bucket and beach towel seem like garish imports from a different register of brightness.

From the beach I take a photograph looking back towards the house. The weather is British, with blowy-grey upside-down clouds. Ev wears a blue shirt and sunhat and his bottom is nude. He crawls away to the left, intent on gouging his truck through the sand, and will not stop until he hits an obstacle. French beachgoers lounge in the background. At the centre of the photo Tom lies asleep in parallel to the lens. Every hour of sleep eases him further away from his encounter with temozolomide. Sleep is so much the best thing for him but lonely for me. I wish he were here. All in black, he lies on his side, his weight on one shoulder, his arms tight crossed. In the photo there is a clear gap of two inches between the sand and his unsupported head. It is a miracle. He is a fakir. The image is proof.

August: We are in a stone house deep in woods in the district bordering the departments of the Lot and the Lot-et-Garonne. A hall, forty feet long, eight wide and large enough to spend time in runs off from the door, with the kitchen facing off the living room and rooms going down opposite each other in pairs. The house sits above a cellar that runs its length and is packed with the tool kit of the second-home: mower, swing, skittles, scythe. It is too hot to move much. At the sun's zenith we pull the shutters each day and the house is made beautifully cool. Tom, Ev and I have come down as the advance party on the train because we cannot drive. Our friends will follow. At the station, which feels like nowhere but is in fact a large town, we are at the casual mercy of the local café owner as to when he might be able to summon a taxi. It is a Saturday night and nothing is being hurried, so I buy milk for Ev and wine for us and Ev plays between the chairs as we sit to wait in the bar. We look like a normal family on holiday.

The house is in an area called Quercy Blanc and the woods are mainly oak, from which the area takes its name, with maple, ash and hawthorn rooted on limestone rock. The taxi climbs into ever more impenetrable woodlands. As we get near, we leave the road and bump down a track lined thick with trees. The driver starts to laugh. *Where the hell is it? Only the English want to hide themselves away so much,* he says. *The English always like to think they are the only ones here. Look at those houses back there,* he shouts, waving his arm; *there are the French, all out in the open, up each other's arses, sticking their noses into each other's pools. The English, they go deep into the woods like hermits. So unsociable*!

The night we arrive, the fields that border the house on three sides are walled with maize. The crop is nine feet high and encloses the house in a live curtain of grain. When Ev is settled in bed we go out to meet it. Each plant is crested with moonlight, fondant and foaming with seeds while the harsh stalks make a black, shifting mass. I imagine it teeming with creatures spying on us beyond our sight. The wind through the stalks generates a moaning that sends us to sleep while its vast bulk absorbs all the other sounds in the valley.

Next morning at seven we wake to an almighty roar. Two huge machines have moved into the field and our horror at the prospect of the breaking of the peace, the thing we have travelled so far to find, is tempered with amazement when we realise that the entire job looks set to be done by noon. Ev is in awe. Humans are mortal but God created machines. By lunchtime the harvesters are done and they knock off, leaving acres of brown stubble razed down to the river. The house we arrived at is now a different one: nude, stranded and exposed to the slope below. The earth, slightly cold at first and strewn with little stones, is scorched within the hour, as if it had always baked like this under the sun and it is impossible to summon up again in the imagination the mystic barrier that surrounded us in the night. When our friends arrive that evening we try to describe it but it makes no sense to them. They see only the rudiments of bare earth met neatly by sky.

The house sits below a road that links the cosmopolitan market town in the valley where you can buy everything with the terse village on the plain that provides milk and eggs. The soundtrack by day is of a billion frogs. By night bats loop on bat zip-wires and a large creature we never see snuffles in the undergrowth, drawn to the kitchen light. Tom and I sit on a bench in the garden to watch the moon melt in an arc below the horizon as fast as ice on a warm hand before we can call the others to witness its exit.

The configuration of our party is four small boys and four adults, one chronically tired. So each day we go for the lines of least resistance: the paddling pool or the Plan d'Eau, playing under the trees or Lego in the sun porch. The nearest I get to my goal of mindlessness is the hammock, so I try to be in it as much as possible. When I can, I turf children off discreetly. Tom has first call on the hammock though. He has first call on everything. There can never be enough sleep. The sleep you get suspended between two trees under light filtered through leaves is a heady one. It is triple-strength, strong as on prescription. In the afternoons the weight of Tom and Ev together takes the hammock so low it crops the top of the grass. Ev lies asleep between Tom's legs and shadows of leaves pattern their bodies like an intricate christening shawl.

One morning at breakfast a lime-green mantis as big as my handspan between thumb and little finger comes to sit on the table. Tom lets it walk up his sleeve and into his hair, where it sits for many minutes to the delight of the little ones. Its companion, an equally large green grasshopper, adopts the oldest and bravest child. Everything is bigger here: bigger, emptier, hotter, drier, quieter and further away. France is giant and it has no one in it. Silence is standard. We can rest.

1.23

There are these simple words that are starting to cause him trouble: *small, single, only, speak, one, tiny, tall, short, sign, slow, same, few, lips, stop, sole, lone*. Tracking elusive words was always Tom's pleasure but now it has added urgency. His recovery is becoming less secure. Out of the blue, pronunciation needs attention. Meaning swoops and flits about and can land on the wrong thing. In a miracle of Tube extension, Kennington Tube becomes Dulwich Tube. Driving through Hackney, a police stakeout becomes police steakhouse. Hand replaces head.

I am a lazy person. His repertoire and verbal sure-footedness was always mine to share. Through him I had access to a store of language: quotes, stories, songs, ideas, poems learned by heart. He has the ability to use the stuff, to turn a phrase, make new. I had thought that learning by heart was the crowning glory of the public school system but maybe he was idiosyncratic even in this. Its worth is clear. Internalisation is power. You know it. It is yours. You can do what you like with it.

Tom's language is our weather, the sky we live under. *Pompholygopaphlasmasin:* this morning he writes this phrase on the blackboard next to our lists and messages in order to find out if he remembers it. He does. *Brekekekex koax koax*, say the chorus of frogs in Aristophanes. It is Monday morning and Ev and me chase round the house being the frogs as I try to get him dressed. It is a dull day and we must find our entertainment indoors. Later, Ev is sitting high above me at Soft Play. He has lost me amidst the apparatus, obscured by netting, coloured balls and ropes. He casts about and sees me below. *Brekekekex koax koax* he says.

In America they call it raising a child. We do not raise, we bring up. It denotes something more like walking alongside with just a hint of correctness. It suggests distance and discipline and a comfortable nearness, as with horses or dogs. In the midst of our disaster I sometimes think, *We must remember to bring him up*. He is not going to stop growing until this firestorm passes. *Rockabye baby/Cradle and crucible.* He is not going to wait or be put on hold. This is it. Zero to three. That's when they say the brain lays down its patterns. Ev is not yet three and it is true. With us he is learning everything he will ever need to know.

His activity is ramping up in pace and speed. He can run off from a standing start shouting over his shoulder and in these moments he is in such ecstasy that although I leap in pursuit, at the same time I will him to go faster. He is a cartoon, a junior league Andy Capp: legs twinkling, feet facing forward, head looking backwards and roaring.

Around London roads is when he most needs discipline but I cannot do this rationally. As soon as I try, anger and anxiety escape me with such force that we are both upturned. The thought that something might happen to Ev, the thing that can happen to children on roads like ours parked tightly with cars along their length, is the trigger. My anger is not commensurate. It is molten and held down in place ever so lightly, like a lid closed with a homemade peg on a billycan set on a campfire. I take the entirety of the thing that is happening to us out on him. Like a coward I attack the smallest and weakest member. I grab him, roar and shout. I am so furious I can hardly see. Why am I angry with no one else? Why just with him? In my childhood, anger was not encouraged. Confrontation best avoided. With whom should I be angry now?

We have come to the National Railway Museum on an extended family outing. It is a vast shed and we are at the limits of our strength. My task is to hold Ev's red anorak in sight as he speeds from train to train. He caresses pistons, walks under safety barriers and rolls himself like a rubber boy behind tender and chassis. The engines are the size of buildings so he is lost in every moment until I catch sight of him again in the next. Tom cannot cope with this. He finds a bench to sit down on. But I can't do it either. When I catch myself in the mirror these days I find it strange that I still operate within a shape, that my body holds its border. I have such fitful energy I feel nausea all the time. I am shrivelled to half my size: the size of a child.

For an hour we spin in low-level pursuit. Aside from the boy in the red coat I don't understand what the other families are doing here. We cannot pretend. Our game is up. What do we want? How shall we proceed? In a pause while Ev wonders where to run to next I grab him and press him to me. I am going to vomit. My head aches and spins. I wish I could die. I think this but by mistake it comes out of my mouth as speech. *No, Mum. Don't die.* He says.

I need things to hit, friends I can scream at. I need meditation, medication, swimming or sex or sleep for months and months and months. I must not say things like that to Ev.

1.24

The air cracks and fizzles. Small energies creel around. I splay my fingers out, stretching them till white flashes between each one. I have been doing this for a year now. I am formulating my response. I am trying to arrive at an intellectual accommodation with death.

What is grief?

I tried to do all my grieving in advance so it might not hurt me later. I tried to burn it up in the firestorm of the initial shock, annihilate it in one pyre. Ash can be dealt with. Take note that this did not work.

What is coping?

This is what it is like: a cave underground deep in rock, hung across its roof with accretions of dripping salts. I am cavernous and hard as mineral. The cave holds a pool of dark water that has not seen light. The water is very cold; it is undrinkable and its size is unmapped. It is mine, but people cannot see it. Only Ev sometimes senses that it is there. All the time people say that I am coping very well. It is impossible to explain my strategy to them. It is opaque even to me.

At a party someone takes my arm and whispers to me, *Strong Woman*. Dear God. My magic vanishes. My power dissolves like powder in water. Weakness is in those nattering companionably all around me. I want please to be one of the weak. The weak are held close and given tea. They are hugged and warmed by the fire. The strong are revered but kept at a distance. They live outside the village.

What is the future?

I imagine I will become different but I don't know how this will come about. My great fear is that I will not be able to achieve difference but will stay the same and be entirely conscious of it.

What is loss?

Loss is a sleeping giant. Moving up the side of an incline I assume it is a mountain or an inert landscape. I have no perspective on the whole. I cannot evaluate its scale but I understand it to be a terrain I must cross and hope that at some point I may gauge its length and breadth. I do not realise that it is not a landscape but a living thing. All knowledge of my situation is physical, gained obscurely by feel through the soles of my feet, palms of my hands and grazes and stumbles on the way. I keep going, tensing my body against the gradient and finding footholds. I feel the surface slip and shift underfoot and its colour and texture is familiar. I wonder why it is warm. I am on it and in it but I have no grasp of what kind of thing it is. I am mapping out its surface by feel and the task entirely absorbs me.

What is happiness?

The same as it was. Happiness does not change.

What is patience?

Patience has no geography. It has no physical border and cannot tolerate an edge or horizon. To even articulate its end or detect the proximity of its limits demands the immediate dissolution of the entire realm. It extends out and out and out. It is a time-based kingdom. It has no other rules.

What is belonging?

The moon pans across the sky. The world spins, the moon one way and the massing clouds pushed by high winds the other. It is a noteworthy moon: perfectly round, fat, big, bright. Our window is its private theatre and tonight we will have a show.

Ev coughs himself awake and I bring him into our bed to watch the drama. *Look at the moon*. He is quiet.

The clouds are like slate cliffs without scale, black with rain. The wind is up now, hysterical, extravagant. It gains momentum as the sky spools from right to left, breathtaking in its speed. It is a bravura motion shot. There are no edit points. Moon, clouds, eyes, triangulate in a sequence lasting many minutes. The moon approaches the edge of the cloud mass. And then, abruptly, before we can prepare ourselves, it exits right and is spun out, free beyond the bulk. The moon stops dead. Without counterpoint to mark its motion it is a perfect disc stranded against unbroken dark. We brake too, stalled and giddy. We are no longer spinning. We three in our location looking up are stilled. Tom sleeps first, then Ev, then me. The room remains bright.

1.25

My American friend Jeff is over and we meet in the local Japanese. About once a year we communicate by email and every four years or so he comes to London. This is a kind of friendship. He has a thin, rough, reddish face, like a plainsman beaten by weather. As he is a film studies lecturer in California this is unlikely. He inhabits the seminar, the lecture hall, the screening room and the library. We met in Hungary, when he appeared in the front row of one of our shows and became one of several Americans en route through Europe that our group befriended. There was usually room in the van for one other with cooking skills or good conversation or both. Jeff is from Indiana and our limited contact has stuck. He says, *So, in spite of Tom's illness you seem to be doing OK.* I reply, *There is nothing in spite of Tom's illness, but yes, we are doing OK.*

Then, as people do, he asks me about my work as an artist. I tell him I am not doing any at the moment and I have no thoughts on the subject. That line of questioning over, and being an academic himself, he asks me about my job. This is easier. I have a part-time post in a university. I teach Art in an Art Department. I find I can continue to do this with ease though I cannot make art and in the months following diagnosis I notice how my attitude to this work subtly changes. The job has shifted its function. It has become recreation. My role in the studio is reactive, and like swimming for a swimmer, the action of swimming incorporates the preparation. Here I can immerse myself in the complex creative worlds of others. We have tutorials, one to one. They bring their secrets. I bring mine. Mine is that it does not matter. In our circumstances this is a blessing.

But I *am* an artist. I have a studio in Bethnal Green. This was where I used to work. In the space of a month after Tom was diagnosed, I sub-let the studio for a year immediately. Recently I have signed for a second sub-let, which means that one calendar year has crossed into another. Over time it seems this can happen, events segue into other events and what drove me then does not motivate me now. I had not believed it possible quite so quickly but I am proof. Today I am here to pick up some papers I have in storage. Just prior to turning the key I am nervous so I stop, wait a bit to get my bearings. Then I open the door and step inside.

It is like being given a capsule to swallow or a strong drink. Memory is as comprehensive and clear as a diagram: of whole seasons of days and hours, through light and night, spent sitting, thinking, planning, making, talking about work, looking at work. A history of all the trails I have ever set in motion lies here, as complex as geological strata. As I breathe in, the warmth of the room unpacks around me. I feel deep affection. I smell it. It is me.

So it *is* me. But on the way my fear was that I might meet my doppelganger – the person who was me and who still would be here had things gone differently. This is the near past. I could argue that it has not been lost but is simply not part of what I am doing now. Why do I not yearn for my life as it was before? Why don't I regret or chafe against its lack? It is not even true that I could get the studio back directly if I wished. We are too volatile. The economy of our household as it stands could not support it.

The studio sits discreetly in a residential area hemmed in by gardens and the backs of terraces. Pigeons peck at the roof and scratch the tiles with deformed feet. Dogs are harassed and bark back and the buzzing of artists' radios filters through the walls. Otherwise it is calm. When I was here I worked usually in silence and these are the sounds I remember. The space is large, high and unheated, so freezing in winter and airless in summer as you might expect. A photographers' light, whitish-grey and perfectly even, sifts down like translucent flour into the room through the window-lantern and two large Velux windows. People liked coming here. It looks like a space you might miss. But I don't. For a year now there has been nothing I wanted to make. The visual world of objects and things, real or proxy on screen, has lost the edge it once had over the rest. The problem is perceptual and cognitive. My compass has shifted. My eyes are looking south, not east, in the direction of home. I have made myself redundant. And if I think back to how I felt before, when I worked here, this fact seems unfathomably remote and dangerous, like an intimate betrayal of self.

Loss of ambition means loss of focus, but the big one is loss of desire. I would have told you, or you might have worked out for yourself, that I was an ambitious person. I was busy. Things were going on. A project, an exhibition, a film, a work, a commission, a residency, a prize: at various points in the recent past, these things were going on. Now they are neither going on nor do I seek them out. I am simply not interested. At one stroke my ambition has gone private and it has a single goal: to keep us as a family alive so that our formation can continue. Our unit of three is like a geometric solid in all its three-dimensional permutations: material, weight, texture, surface, patina, form, colouration. This is all the matter I can grasp in my hands.

That this ambition is concrete yet different from any I have ever held before is a stark fact. I cannot achieve my ambition by my own or any other ends. By hard work I cannot make it happen, by being good I cannot make it happen, by self-sacrifice I cannot make it happen, by being clever I cannot make it happen, by being more creative I cannot make it happen. My previous ambitions, reliant on skill and will, are rendered mute, inert, of no interest.

So not to have any ideas at all, not for objects or images or films, seems to be the end of me. More singular still is not to care. But it is a fantastical, wilful abandonment. Not to choose is incredible. It makes the end of me so beautifully slight. I have an imperative. I may resist the imperative or I can love the imperative, it makes no difference. By no effort of will can I change the terms. All I can do is change my approach.

Standing in the doorway of the studio picking out the scents of shavings and glue, dust, papers, heat trapped under plastic and old tea, I am smiling. Relieved. Everything is in order. Aside from being with Ev and Tom, all I can do is put one word down after another and rearrange them so that you might have a sense of what they mean. This is the work and it seems endeavour enough. I am almost content.

1.26

The smallest things have the greatest mass.

Travelling is a risk. Going anywhere is a risk, so you could argue that we may as well be in Spain. We go to Madrid.

A flat white cloud like a neat child's drawing outlined in blue hangs over the city. We are at the Prado. Inside the air is serene. Mid-week crowds move evenly in a herd-daze. We have come to see the Goya rooms, where the full-length canvases show uneasy courtiers and sullen kings waiting for the republic to hit them like a rain of eggs and rotten fruit. From afar I see a tiny painting, more potent than anything in the room. The picture is called *Vuelo de Brujas*, The Flight of the Witches, and it's from 1798. I touch his sleeve and pull him over.

A man runs towards us, blinded by a sheet covering his head. Behind him on the left lies another man foreshortened on the shallow ground. He is in despair. His stops his ears and wants neither to hear nor see what is going on. The foreground is a strip of sand and the background noir speeds on to it soaking it up like a blotter. To the right stands a donkey, daft as a lever. The donkey's head and skinny neck jut into the painting and its baggy nose grazes the edge of the sand. Flying above are three witches, their limbs plaited together like an airborne puzzle or pretzel. They are carrying a third man who is struggling for his life. What will they do to him? No good. Their faces are intent and shadowed, impossible to read.

The witches are naked to the waist. Their tall split-spire hats of pink, yellow and blue meet in an apex at the top of the painting as they attend to their charge. Their flight is articulate and self-generated: weights and lights and stresses fall precisely for their height and position in the air. How did he imagine this? Unlike most human fliers in paintings, they are not pretending to fly. This is a record of what three witches would look like if they bore aloft another person in order to destroy him.

1.27

An ivory sap obscures my vision. I have conjunctivitis. It is viscous and tough and hangs Christmassy on the lashes. My eyes are rimmed red and suctioned hard into my face. The diagnosis is the same from every layman I meet: *Run down. Run down*. I have an ulcer and spend two nights mostly awake unable to swallow without pain. It feels oddly exhilarating and super-charged, as if the possibilities are finally becoming limitless. Maybe I can live even without sleep.

We are a mess. For a while our night is continuous with our day and as disorganised; people rising, squalling, coughing, swapping beds, getting drinks – hot milk with turmeric – watching children's DVDs in bed. All the while outside it snows, an early-year fall, intermittently hard and soft but deep. Snow piles up and blends all edges, softening the residential streets and gardens and anointing the roofs of cars like risen cakes perfectly baked. If it weren't for the pain there's a fizzy anarchy about. We are characters crammed into an apartment in a Russian novel, complicit in the plot that binds our fates together, doing acts of kindness for each other and groaning and cursing all the while. My driving test is cancelled under the snow. Tom has another scan and it is *Good*. On the far side of the world an earthquake shakes Haiti to rubble.

Since the middle of last year I have been learning two new skills, driving and swimming, both means of propelling myself forward.

I was always uneasy in water, suspicious. I clung to the sides, hugged the steps and shallows and my toes were programmed to feel for the bottom. Now this changes. I learn to put my head beneath the surface and keep my weight low, face to the floor. I discover the glide and visualise the top of my head aiming forward as if pulled on a line of the thinnest, purest, soluble fibre from the other end of the pool. My lung capacity, through years of singing and brass instruments, is large. I can breathe long and glide long and I practise an ultra slow, streamlined action. I am given my first pair of goggles and suddenly I can see underwater. Why did no one show me this before? I feel cheated. With these eyes I dip to the bottom like a pearl diver to finger the smooth tiles and gauge with my body the volume of the pool. Its pearl-white grid is as elegant as a submerged dance hall, an inverted jewel in a municipal shell. I swim a length underwater coming up only once with hardly a ripple. I have not done a pool-length for years. At school I swam like a sewing machine in a dotted line of ragged splashes, each splash marking a small drowning.

Learning to drive is more pressing, as Tom's diagnosis meant that he had to stop. On the road I learn a system of movements by heart until they become my own. Throughout the winter and into the New

Year I roll in a sort of dream around the curls and traffic snags of south London; low-rises in creams and browns and greys splashed with tatty brick. Charity shops, speed humps, cemeteries, one-way systems, schools, chicanes, housing estates, markets, roundabouts, bus lanes, dead-ends: I spin on, pausing only to turn on three points of an ill-drawn triangle or reverse, prim and staid, around a corner. I love changing gear; my eyes and brain are fixed to the task and for the duration of the lesson I am free: West Wickham, Elmers End, Croydon and Crystal Palace, Woodside, Eden Park, Norwood and Anerley. Once, in a piece of late-year optical evening magic, I crested a hill to see a giant orange sun swollen three times as big as normal hanging below me over the Kingdom of the South. I have never been to these places and I will never come to them again. This is my wish.

The fixed agenda of the car muffles and shushes me. Padded leather absorbs anxiety and the magic tree is a placebo. I do not need to sob in front of the instructor. I see him twice a week but I never speak of what is going on. As the snow melts I pass with a reverse arabesque that parks me so sweetly I exhale an audible hiss of delight and exchange eyes with the tester. I am a driver.

One Saturday morning about a week later I am on the road encased in my new status. I park and practise sitting in the car like others do with my chin leaning on my arm at the open window and my gaze loose and idle like a dog. The radio is on and the weak sun has sent Ev to sleep in the back. The skin on my arm is warming. A man – *a bad driver* – grinds his wheel against the wheel of a stationary car as he negotiates the tight-parked street. Couples curl in sync into their cars and drive off in flawless motion without signalling at all. A woman clacks past me with shopping. This is my gift to myself. I see all of it and none of them see me. I am in a car therefore I am invisible. I am at home in all the cars of my childhood. I am just like everybody else.

1.28

It is February but the future has arrived early. Tom has a severe fit in the small hours of the morning. He had gone away by himself to get some writing done in a house by the sea and was due home today. It is evening, he is back with us, lying down quietly upstairs. He can talk after a fashion, read a little but he can't write. He is estranged from himself.

We phone each other countless times as a matter of course – this was always our habit – and so unable to reach him throughout the day I knew that something was wrong, but while waiting for him to call me, come home or do anything comprehensible, my insides turn to paste and I shit myself on the way home from nursery.

The walk from nursery is the daily setting for Ev's grand narratives. It is the chance for his imagination to revisit afresh the cracked world of the pavement, inspect each drain, gate, pile of leaves, parked car or whatever catches his eye along the way. It lasts forever. Desperate, I clamp down on his indulgences and haul him on as he halts at pretend stoplights or level crossings and balks at kerbs as if they were cliffs. From the staff I hear that he has been ebullient and hyperbolic, ramming the other children with his body like a daft goat. Some children do this as standard but Ev does not. His behaviour has gone wonky this week with Tom away. It's not that serious, just a shade off beam from his usual sunny engagement, but it throws me. All must love him. Everyone must be his friend. He needs them even more now than if his father were going to last forever. I am alert to every nuance of his behaviour as I understand him to be alert to every nuance of ours. If I could make a wish for him, it would be that that the pristine selfishness of childhood would wrap him in multiple layers like clingfilm, proof him and seal him up one hundred per cent. I would wish him *impenetrability*. I know this is not how it works. This is not a good-fairy wish. Ev is alive to the world uncensored. His interest doesn't stop at ants or plastic dinosaurs but roams intelligently round us like a data tracker programmed throughout waking hours: noticing, registering, following, collecting, finding, piecing together and storing information. When I pick him up today, *I need my daddy* is the first thing that comes out of his mouth and it is a just complaint. I had told him that we would come to fetch him from nursery together. That was the plan. But Tom is somewhere in the vacant stretch between London and the south coast, past the Isle of Sheppey, on to Thanet, Kent and the sea. He is not answering the phone so I have no way of finding out where he is.

Tom at the coast and in the aftermath of the fit retains the fact that he had meant to buy seafood to bring home to us this evening. Roll-mop he can name as *roll-map* but the word *crab* escapes him. Before leaving the house where he is staying, he thinks about the idea and image of a crab for a long time. He draws a picture of it in his notebook, as if summoning its image would render the associated word. Finally, after

I don't know how long or in what order, the word either surfaces or the lack of it recedes. He arrives at *crab* and goes out to the stall to make the purchase. The pursuing of normality especially where it intersects with pleasure is a matter of pride. Much later he hands me the fresh, dressed crabmeat, brown and white, and from a far, far distance I salute his tenacity, his practical intelligence, his cool.

Around five o'clock he manages to call me but he is incoherent. I have a friend with a car on standby to go and look for him but he cannot frame the words to tell me where he is. His language has the bones of meaning but not much beyond. So he navigates to the station and finds the train and in London somehow gets a taxi to bring him home. On arrival at Victoria Station he sees the words Victoria St. What does St mean? He thinks Saint but understands this to be wrong in context. Incredibly he works it out by looking at a map, a complex pictorial scheme for a foreigner to interpret at the best of times. Rd for road. Ave for avenue. Finally, St comes, for station. Later he describes all this to me easily. In his pocket he has one of the cards we made with his name and address, numbers for him and me, and a note saying that he is having a focal fit and the finder of him might helpfully contact me. He doesn't think of any of this and doesn't use the card.

At work throughout the day I feel the force of his absence and the measure of the distance between us, though it took hours to work out that something serious was wrong. *He might have worked so late he slept through the morning. He may be on his way home already.* All these reassurances, this rationalising, the many things one can think. My patterns of alertness to him move fast. They are so fickle and mobile that it is hard to describe their movements but at root there is the understanding that something is always wrong. How wrong is the fluctuant that flows from the root. Like the force of a wave, it might be a gentle ripple or it could be the crash that drowns and takes all.

If you imagine a hole in the sea and the energy required to maintain it, it might be a bit like this. Barry Flanagan came up with this idea, *A Hole in the Sea,* first as a print and then as a video in 1969. His conception looks anodyne in itself: serene. But it allows you into such a phenomenon. You can imagine the rim of a hole in the sea as the most untenable place in the universe, an impossible stop in a perfect continual broil seething with supernatural force. Of course it would not be a hole but a tube. A tube is a hole all the way down. In *Fantasia,* the Magician banishes the waters in great cymbal crashes, forcing apart dramatic crests of white cartoon spume. Charlton Heston as Moses in *The Ten Commandments* worked through exhortation and fear to lead his people through the sea. His waters don't dare to close until he allows. The parting creates a neat edge, like a celluloid trench dug with a spade.

For Tom to be at home is perfectly normal. He works at home and the things he needs for his work are mostly near at hand. But when he is away from me as he must be sometimes and not within easy reach, say on a train going to an exhibition or visiting a friend out of town, it is as if I am maintaining a hole in the sea. An impossible, solid shape held by psychic force all the way down, with millions of cubic metres of water pressing in ready to close it. The pressure is that something should happen when I am not there. But the pressure is the same even if nothing happens. Days mostly go perfectly well. That nothing should happen on a given day is only luck. The situation is paradoxical. He is still ill.

SECTION 2

2.1

27 March 2010

Dear Friends

We haven't sent out one of these messages since last July. Tom has had a scan every three months since then. Last week there was another. This time the news was bad. The tumour has started to grow, and another course of treatment is needed. We don't know exactly what it will be, but some kind of chemotherapy, starting in about a fortnight.

Tom feels mainly well but is having some fits and minor speech problems. His writing continues well. Ev is gorgeous and very nearly three. Marion has just passed her driving test. But all is immediately uncertain. The next months of treatment are going to be difficult. So we say again how important it is to us that our friends are in touch. Please do write, phone, text, email, visit, invite, come for dinner.

We look forward to hearing from you.

With love

Spring. There is going to be destruction: the obliteration of a person, his intellect, his experience and his agency. I am to watch it. This is my part. There is no deserving or undeserving. There is no better and no worse. Cold has pained the ground for months. Now the garden is bursting and splitting. From the window each morning I mark the naked clay ceding to green. I am against lyricism, against the spring, against all growth, against all fantasies, against all nature. Blast growth and all things that grow. It is irrelevant, stupid, a waste. As nature is indifferent to me, so am I to it.

As the air outside thickens and the warmth encourages the earth to release its smell, something is starting to go wrong. It is now March. I say it is March the eleventh. In one week, Tom will have another scan. This is the one to fear.

Today as he stands mid-morning by the kettle chatting and making tea, his language trips into rhythmically correct nonsense. It is ludic, quickly recoverable, but it does not sit either with fits or with his usual verbal slippages and we note the difference in its texture immediately. It is as if language problems are self-seeding and taking root elsewhere. The primary confusions up till now have been in epileptic shocks of greater or lesser intensity. Some lie under the radar, barely registering. Others are brash. He is silenced and cannot frame a sentence with meaning. When this happens, the thought that no sense will ever be made again is visual like a solid mass, as real as an object is real, a tin or a plate or a pen. For him it is different. Fear is not the issue. Even in the thick of it he is always trying to work out what is going on, to test himself. He is his own best monitor. There have not been so many fits, but outside them complexity is multiplying and thousands of lesser confusions also occur. Words slip out, switches are stumbled over and substitutions made. Like exotic fauna the varieties of language proliferate.

The scan results are as expected. After nine months of post-chemo stasis it is springtime. The tumour is growing again.

Spring. *Magnolia soulangeana* opens its bells and we are well. Normality is gifted in the form of steroids, 2mg daily, and immediately he tightens his grip on language and on the connection of meaning to word. He feels much stronger, stimulated. He can do simple tasks without exhaustion: pick up Ev and carry him. How we adore this high false peak. It lasts quite a short time, but time is a material stream and we never know how long it will last so we are taken in by it, of course we are. We are as ever in the moment and we are well – so we are forever well. We are not sanguine but we have been here before. We are doing our work and we know what the work is. We know we are good at it. We splash about like birds in a birdbath.

2.2

10 April 2010

Dear Friends

Since our last news at the end of March, things have moved very quickly. The surgeon has now looked at the scans, and recommends another operation. It is lucky that the tumour is growing back in the same place, on the edge of the brain. Tom will be going into Queen Square hospital on Monday, and the operation will be on Tuesday 13 April. The procedure is very similar to the last one, with the same surgeon and we hope it is as successful. It is all extremely short notice. Tom will be out of action now for an uncertain period.

This is a time of great stress for us. Offers of help, practical, emotional, culinary, comradely, or otherwise enlivening – all will be gratefully received. If we don't get back to you immediately don't worry.

We should say how much your support and contact so far has meant to us three. Thank you.

With love

The consultants go into conference and within days they come up with a plan. We mark the speed at which they move. Tom is to have another operation. This was not expected. Most people don't get a second shot at the knife. Some cells that escaped and were not excised during the first operation are growing again, but rather than burrowing deep into the thinking part they are heading towards the surface like plants to light. This makes them accessible to the blade. *The Thinking Part* – have I actually learned anything in all this time? Tom wants to be treated like an organism and this attitude serves him well. Together we keep ourselves in joint ignorance of biology beyond the basics. A school textbook would do as well.

I feel a fraud. Because I am the authority, I am always given the last word in any conversation with the laity. But I don't have so many words. The extent of my knowledge might begin and end in one speech. On the spot I can stall and run out of facts. I might talk freely about Temodal or chemo implants but should someone quiz me further I would spin out softly into vagueness or make it up. We repeat like clever little parrots what we are told by this or that consultant and we try so hard to hold on to the wording and inflection as we pass the news on to others. We are like children bewitched, using words as spells or charms, as if our lives depended on these tokens of correctness of form or tone of voice.

This conscious care and the desire not to embellish has the force of an ideological position. We hold that it's important to communicate the situation and our attitude to it without bias, false hope or scope for misunderstanding. We try not to skew the dialogue and keep the words free of inflection. We are trying to spare ourselves something so that by extension others may be spared.

This goes spectacularly awry in an early conversation with Dr B. I am not present and Tom is clearly drifting. He comes away with the morsel that something is shrinking. *Something, what thing? Some part. What? Some bad part. The area of the tumour? The tumour bed? The surround? The edge? The rind. The rind? Can it really be the rind?* We never discover what the word she used was or what it meant but it does not seem to matter. After this when Dr B phones, we take her calls jointly. She speaks to him and then to me and afterwards we repeat the whole conversation again to each other, examining the texture of the words for flaws as we say them aloud in our own voices.

There is a pattern to these things and how we handle them. At dusk we go into the garden. It's a good place to talk, standing against the blank fall of the back of the house, beneath Ev's window where he sleeps. First we stand opposite each other close up. Then we turn to face the house side-by-side, our shoulders touching. Plants crowd round, their colours drained. Artemisia flares in the half-light. Abutilon blurs its bells. Another operation means another visit to Mr K. We have an appointment already. I had not thought I would be seeing him again.

It is Friday. Mr K is in blue scrubs and soiled white crocs. He seems younger than he did before, though I have no idea of his age. He may be younger than me: strange how these things matter. Now that he is intimate with Tom, having gone once already inside his brain, his manner is easier with us. I listen hard to everything he says. I have a pencil to write things down but it is a prop and I do not use it. My memory of these conversations is very accurate.

Mr K has a vision. It is a precise field. He works first with the visual picture – the MRI – and he has a developed knowledge of what its fuzzy, amorphous tones and areas of grey segueing into darker grey might mean. There are limits to this. An MRI is a monochrome, ill-defined image; it resembles a photocopy but if anyone can interpret it, it is he. He has good tools, a good team, a good hand and an exquisite sense of mass and space. He is a craftsman. What else might he do: lace-work, restoring veneers, model-making? Maybe he goes for risk. Perhaps he skis or likes to jump off tall buildings. I doubt this. I know two things about him. He is careful and he is confident. The brain is not so big. In a tight space he is astute. He understands the layout where the tumour sits and what occurs immediately around and behind, deeper into the brain. Cut to one side for speech, to the other for emotion, back a bit for anger. This is his domain. We are his guests.

If the conversation strays from the visual or the factual, his lack of interest is ever so faintly and minutely signalled. I try to work out how the signal goes: a slight breath, a shift, a nostril flares, his mouth marginally puckers, a muscle in his leg adjusts itself. This occurs when we introduce narrative. Narrative means symptoms. Symptoms mean the description of how this thing affects us in daily life. Tom finds this comforting. On the scale of things, his expertise outweighs our anecdote.

He says it would not be logical not to operate and would we like to do it on Tuesday? We nod. We would like to do it on Tuesday. We don't need to look in the diary. We have nothing else that could compete. *Good.* He commits us to the system with perfect ease, efficiency and courtesy. *I shall make a phone call to my friend Fred.* We are entered, and over the next hour, height, blood, heart, chest, weight, pressure, all are taken down and stickers stuck on dozens of samples. Tom's name is asked over and over. Tom's name is written over and over.

We are at the slippery point that defines the whole game. We are embodied. Consciousness must have a shape. The brain can be pictured. It has mass, weight, size, geography. It has history. Like any country, events can happen in it that can be plotted spatially. These local events can be identified, studied, and can determine the whole. This means the real, whole, whole – whether Tom will have the use of memory to think of a poem, use of understanding to determine which lines to recall, use of sensibility to play with words and form them into significant shapes, use of humour to make jokes, use of tact to know when not to make them, use of sense to make a choice, take a measure, use of motor to cross a road, cook an egg, use of speech to reveal himself and *all this* to us. *All this* has a physical root. *All this* is matter. *All this* is here endangered. *All this* is the business of Mr K.

So at the weekend, the day before our second entry into hospital for brain surgery, we have a party to celebrate the third birthday of Ev. Seven little children are invited and two dozen adults. It is a gorgeous day. Tom in the garden prepares the games. He paints a solid stumpy donkey on a bit of board for Pin the Tail and stuffs a sock for Splat the Rat. In the kitchen the table is laid with food: sausages, chicken, hummus, Hula Hoops, carrot, apple juice, pots of wine. The birthday cake is Ev's choice, tiers of cream and strawberries. It is a very good party. Pass the Parcel goes to the tune from *The Dambusters*. Ev sleeps through the manic preparations in his buggy and rises fresh to the event with the arrival of the first guests as is his due. Sharing is ordained. Snatching, biting and pinching are proscribed. Tears are limited. It is all quite simple. Everyone is very happy. The birthday is maximal. It could not have been otherwise.

2.3

Tuesday 13 April brings a wound, a river and a mistake: all the hallmarks of tarot casting or bad omen. Early on I realise that things are going against me. By 8 a.m. I have crossed the river twice already, to the hospital once for a kiss, then south again to deal with Ev. In the material traffic across different registers and scales of importance, the smaller details – the child, the hospital, the logistics of the city – collide with the major ones: the operation is at eight and I am afraid.

Ev is sent away. Over and over I deliver him into the arms of others. That he is the child he is allows me to do this without pause. But something is wrong above the conscious anxiety I am feeling, a kind of rigidity, a meta-ache I cannot place. It must be mine, for where else could it exist that I might feel it, but it seems separate, extending outside me like a zone apart. Waiting for Ev to go, I count the seconds until I can stop being his mother. Poor Ev. He is not fooled. What mother wears dark glasses indoors and does not kiss goodbye? As soon as he is gone I break like a dry stick. I am shaking violently, not myself. I recognise the high, repeated wailing to be my own voice but it too seems separate. It ascends, breaks, squeaks, mutes. It is pitiful. But I have done this before, this operation. I should be OK. I have done this before.

My friend is with me and she does not leave my side. She feeds me sugar in tea and fat and salt in bacon and butter but I am overrun. Demons swarm at my head and in my ears. I have no fight left and give in to their idiot murmuring. They whisper that he will die. They say that I will lose him.

The Thames lies between us. It marks the divide between home and hospital and in the course of the day I cross it six times from south to north and north to south as if under compulsion. Miscommunication and incoherence drive the action of the day forward. The silver river is our test and task. I notice it afresh each time and it hurts me afresh each time. The water is serpentine, obscenely bright under the sun, and pressed along its bank, the geometric solids of the City: domes, towers, blocks, spires and wheel refract light in sentinel beams that send codes up into the sky. What do they say? They say he will die. They say today is our last day.

At the hospital we wait. Where I don't know but it is hours – two? More? Then I get a message that Tom is still in theatre. This makes no sense. Craniotomy Number Two is simple brain surgery. It is a straightforward procedure and he should have been out well before now. We do not know what to do or what to think but moving is a surrogate for doing and thinking so we get in a taxi and head for home. I call friends around me in advance of disaster. My finger pokes at their numbers but I don't know what it is I am asking. To hear my voice, to be near, prepare. *What if he dies*? I am not ready.

Then, nearing home, we get another call. No, in fact he got out some time ago. He is doing well. He has asked me to call him. He is waiting for me. The first message was only wrong. It was simply a mistake and no significance should be attached to it. Back we go in convulsion, back across the river.

All the time, in cars and corridors, I cannot stop shaking. I am wrapped in coats but there is not warmth enough in the sun. The sequence of the day is irrational. There is nowhere to go. The waiting room has nowhere to wait and the only place I need to be is lying down. Each hour elongates beyond use, yet each is so dense I can't understand how we move only one digit on at a time. At some point, I don't know when, before or after what, we are in the families' room. It is a tiny galley space filled with women from an extended Asian family. Their relative is in trouble and they do not believe he will live. They unwrap great oblongs of sandwiches in silver foil and settle down.

Another time, I lie for an hour in a friend's bed high above the street. Why is it so quiet? The cars funnelling at ground level seem to lose their force and by the time it reaches the fourth floor the noise is aerated. Silence damps the rowdy demons at last. I am struck with love for her bed. I do not pay my bed any attention and it returns the lack. Mine is the bed of a married person, stained with tea and child-wee. Hers is white and comely, with pillows and bolsters and proud and proper stuffing. It seeks to hold me and I long to rest but something is wrong. Anxiety seeps like a chemical stain on to her sheets. Am I hallucinating? I check the bed over and over for brown fluid. Why can't I see it? But it seems I do sleep for fragments of an intermittent hour and when I wake, my phone is ringing. I can go and see him.

Out of the voodoo chronicle of the day the real story shapes itself slowly. It has been nothing like what I have experienced but another sort of time entirely. My terrors have been of the river and the swamp: airborne and infectious, not grounded. My day is a neurotic parallel of Tom's. In the real world, everything has been efficient and routine. All has been done hygienically well. The schedule has gone to plan. The news is practical, robust, good-hearted and standard. It might be written in bold red pen on a whiteboard. That Tom is well. The operation has been good. The tumour has been debulked. Next to his name would be a box drawn with a smiley face.

In the late afternoon somewhere towards the end of the long sequence, I find him in the Recovery Room and when I do he is wholly himself, sitting up in the ward, wildly impatient and raging to talk. *Where have you been?* His head has a comedy bandage. He is lucid, happy, bored and ready to go. I have no idea at all how to communicate what has just happened or how to correlate it with his new-minted face or the tumbling words that signal the continuing presence of his Own True Brain. I am speechless, ecstatic, stupefied and ground to dust. My mouth opens and shuts on the hinge of my jaw. I taste metal on my tongue. Where have I been?

After the whole twelve hours is done, leaving only its rock-hard, raw, salt trail on me that I won't shake off for weeks, friends bring me home to bed to shiver under piles of blankets. Ev comes back very late. This is the last episode. I have a virus and he has it too. He vomits on the bedroom carpet beside me.

2.4

13 April 2010

Dear Friends

The operation went well. Tom is sitting up, talking, eating, reading. He looks extremely good. All praise to the surgeon.

With love

In a bold pre-emptive move the volcano Eyjafjallajökull erupts into the air and from this catalyst many things follow. Across much of northern Europe people stop flying. Not in mid-air, though you might think this from the commotion. They remain afar, wherever they happen to be, and as the days pass clamour ever louder to be brought home. The volcano cannot be appeased so they turn their fire on systems and institutions. Marriages are missed, reconciliations delayed, families already stressed are strained further. Inconvenience is the sorriest disaster.

The air above Iceland has an impossible forever-and-ever clarity. It is storybook air: sheer up and up and higher and higher. Glassiness distorts and tricks the far into seeming near, as if you could whisper to someone miles away yet never see their eyes light up to hear you. Years ago, I set out to pat the dark snout of the glacier Vatnajökull across a stubby terrain of moss, stalked and dive-bombed by gulls. After an hour of walking it remained like an illusion the same size and distance away from me. When I finally reached it, I stayed only minutes and wanted to turn back as if I had been mistaken. I was embarrassed and pretended I hadn't wanted to see it really. It was a dripping, moaning mass of vertical water: the abyss, beached and landlocked, an appalling creature. Blue like a sea brewing a storm, green as kelp and beyond filthy, it seemed unspeakable. Too many categories of phenomena were conflated. My brain didn't like it.

Ev confuses ash with gas but understands about planes and is very interested in this development. We follow the unfolding northern saga on the radio from the bed. I am flattened, wiped out. For recreation I have two squares of visible window air. Both are blocked out with sky and empty so I register directly the lack of travel above my territory.

Tom is in hospital recovering well from surgery. Ev is covered in rash, not ash or gas. We are both infectious so neither he nor I can visit him.

When I phone, he sounds wildly cheerful. I hear of pies, soups, snacks and company supplied to his bed by a tag-team of friends. I am jealous. He has a small aphasic fit, witnessed expertly by Dr Matt, our neurologist friend, who neatly updates the patient's notes in person.

The bedside of a man in hospital can be staged as comedy or drama, with both colliding at any moment. The play's context, like sickness or wellness, is embodied in the patient. Different aspects of a narrative enter and exit, cross and meet, in combinations that may be disastrous or felicitous. Here, the mother and the father who do not speak may fetch up together or the implacable grudge-bearer might find his ancient target sitting smug among the peaches. Friends from different spheres can exchange numbers and fall in love. The unwelcome may cloud the visit. Or – no one may come at all. That must surely be the most fearful of shows.

It is now five days since the operation on Tom's brain and he can still speak to me. Joy. The air is holding its breath. The sky is ultra-blue: no contrails, no clouds, no sound, no low-flies, no disturbances of any kind anywhere. Birds are taking over. Soon it will be all birds. It is an epic time, momentous like the medieval moon at eclipse. Rivers will run red and the harvest will lie down in the fields. Two-headed lambs will be born. For the generations who have tasted the drug of flight, this has never happened and we who are not stuck in airports or waiting for others to return to us like it very much. On it continues, the great grounding, starting on the Thursday, on through Friday, Saturday, Sunday and into the next week. All over that long, long weekend everyone is attached to the earth. I hold the ground under my feet and my physical grasp of it as near divine. This is bliss.

We live in a slowed-down part of one of the biggest, fastest cities on earth. The day has been perfect. It is nearly nine in the evening. From my bed I watch the sky's incremental bands: dark, deep, pale, wan, white, gold, slide separate into each other. The moon is a crisp paper-cut. The air is silent but for birds. Nothing. It is wonderland. He has survived. I have survived. Ev has survived. We are not unchanged. We are scathed.

2.5

22 April 2010

Dear Friends

Tom is back home and feeling well. We are all happy to be together again.

More chemo is now expected soon. Thanks for your support. We look forward very much to seeing you.

With love

On Firle Beacon the air is opaque, impossibly fine and laced with water in sequin patterns. Spray shimmies into our mouths from every angle and we drink from source. Ahead, the path snakes into silver and the land on either side slopes away part-hid. No one else is here. It is too windy, too wet. Black-headed sheep clump around the croppy bushes and rocks. Their wool is scuffed and dirty, stuck with bracken and bits of gorse. The ground is uneven, littered with stones and the remains of cairns, and sand-coloured grasses shelter in the hollows. The wire fence that edges the path is twined with wool an exact match of the sky. Frenetic all along its length, it is alive with every gust.

Ev runs away from me shouting towards the sheep and his body veils with rain to almost nothing. Even though I know they will not charge him, I gauge the hard mask of their faces, their yellow teeth and filthy hooves against his softness. He runs directly into the sheep camp, causing them to up and lumber off a few metres distance: bored, blank, thunderous. I yell at him. *Stop. Come back.*

I do not think, *This is the last time we will do this*. It does not enter my head. The will to the future is too strong, stronger than this. Air and rain and wind whirl around us. We are at the intersection of all the energy on the high path and we take it up into our bodies. Our clothes are pearls. We are made luminous with pearls. The corners of my open mouth are wet and my voice shines against the wind as I shout in Tom's ear. *We must come here again. We will walk this way. We will come here again.*

2.6

It is the twenty-first of June. We have hit the mid-point. Today the year turns on itself and begins its retreat to narrow, weak hours of daylight folded into slabs of darkness. This year the ebb has greater urgency than the flow. I can feel its pull already. Bob our neighbour comes round. Through the frosted glass in the door I see him standing sentry holding what looks like a pastel-coloured hat. It is a plate with a bowl upturned on it and underneath that an exemplary cake, made by his daughter at catering college: three tiers of cream and a neat top packing of blueberries. This is great. Holed up in our private and eventful space we are feeling abandoned and alone, so this small incursion is worth more than its weight in cake. To keep our friends by us, we need to keep them informed and when there is nothing really to tell them, we stop. Most of the time, between scans played out in intervals of three months, we are waiting to see what is going to happen and what is there to say about that? So we say nothing.

But saying nothing is not the same as feeling nothing. We are very fragile and we can feel quickly forgotten. There is no way to balance these competing stresses, to make a life like ours work. Sustaining the precise amount of attention we need from the outside world evenly and forever is not something that is in my power.

Tom has some strategic aim in mind regarding the displacement of books. Since he came back from hospital he is moving the library around a lot, parking things in different places and shifting sections en bloc. I'm not quite sure why he is doing this but I suspect it is to do with solidity and the reinforcement of each category. They are like bricks. He is making our walls impermeable and hence shoring up his recall. Books make us another house again. We have 118m of shelving. I know because I built them. All of them are full. Our living space is 5 per cent smaller because of books. Shelves cover both walls in the hall, one from floor to ceiling, fill two sides of one bedroom entire and both sides of the fireplace in the living room. One side of another bedroom is books and so is the upper end wall in the light well, though this can be reached by ladder only. It is not an equal split. A ragged portion a few metres wide is mine. The rest is Tom's. He is a bibliophile. Buying books is his habit. Reading them is his work and life.

His spatial memory remains acute and when he needs to look something up he always remembers exactly where the book is that he might need, upstairs or down, and on what shelf. More wondrous still, he can remember what quote is in what book and where it lies. Only now often it is me who reads it.

I have been unable to read since this began and it is getting worse. My eyes can't focus, they skit across, landing on words and skimming them for meaning as if they were simply a platform for something else more important. Fiction is impossible. Why would you want to make anything up? Newspapers are nearly too difficult. I stare at the spines in the hall wondering if I should open one. Will they be of help? I have heard it said that books can help in dark times but I don't do it. In my heart I doubt it.

The disparity between us in reading has broadened. His speech can still be very good so this is not always detectable. You might register only an undertow of disquiet, a ripple in the sense and order of things. He is back at work. It takes more time but always comes out right. But the more words slip away, the more it matters to him to know what they are, while I hardly read them at all. More precisely, I read the ones he needs to use. We are ever elastic. Within our stretch, what one lacks the other makes up. My lack is temporal and selective. The reason I do not read is because words are irrelevant. They become relevant when he needs them. I can see the ones he is looking for. I can help him find them. If he is chasing something, I know it. I always find it, read it back for him and he understands it perfectly. No other words exist. I have stopped using my eyes. I think with his.

Since coming home there are fresh difficulties. He has trouble saying the name of the hospital or the name of the friend who came yesterday. He calls me to the study where he is looking up something in the thesaurus. The word is *disaster*. *They can't have got rid of it!* he says. *Maddening*! As he has spelled it *distaster,* he cannot find it. Physically there is a lot of strain. Weakness and muscle failure is starting to sting him and creep again around the joints, fingers and calves and in parts of his arms. This is steroids at their warring work. Pain seeks out the interstices where uncertain seams of deep tissue meet, a side effect from first increasing and then cutting down on steroids, but the speech trouble is a major worry. A friend asks me, with reference to our financial future or strategic thinking, if I am delaying putting any plans in place until the crisis hits. Hits? How will we know when crisis hits? It is all crisis. It is a stick of solid rock with the letters C-R-I-S-I-S all the way through. We just do not know its length.

Money is a worry. I will set it out here as sometimes in the middle of the night it presents itself to me. We don't know what will happen. Tom earns money as a writer. How long will he continue to earn? When will it stop? What will happen when it does? In the beginning I would wake soaked in such a sweat of ice it needed changes of sheets. Sweat is the main reaction my body has to crisis: Atlantic and Pacific quantities, estuaries and whole pools stream out of me. I am an icon that weeps all over its skin: a marvel to be exhibited and worshipped. I shall gather a sect of the faithful to devote their lives to me as keepers, making tea, burning incense, stroking and wiping down my long glistening surface with chamois and charging an entry fee. I need to earn money. I shall make people pay to look at me.

Feebly I start up conversations. We need to talk about provision, strategies, savings, but this has never been our ambit. We are much too late. We have no debts bar our home but we do have to continue living. This is what drowns me in the night. There are agencies I can talk to, Macmillan, Citizens Advice, forms I can fill in, and I do. When I have time and volition I do. But Tom has no interest in these conversations. His concerns are not these. This is so understandable that I abandon my case. His living depends on speaking and writing and when he cannot speak and write then his income, the main of our two, is gone. Overnight our household is unsustainable. I will be the sole earner and carer to both. My earning power has been undermined this last year to such a degree I can't bring myself to look at it.

But sitting hard by this question is a critical one that casts the other into shade. If Tom lives for a long time as a person who depends on speaking and writing and he cannot speak or write, then where is Tom? If you hear this, tell me.

Ev and I go out to the pools and lidos of London. There is no greener city this year. Trees and water, water and trees, with a hard dappled light bouncing between is where the children like to gather in bright, hot sun. The paddling pool in the park is the watering-hole for all the locals. Adults stand in groups as overseers, mid-calf in water, arms folded. Those with older children have a policy of minimal intervention or feign lack of interest. Those with younger ones will not miss a single splash. They hover enraptured, their eyes never leaving their young.

Kids steam about: naked, in pants, T-shirts, every kind of swimsuit and school uniform soaked on to their bodies. Babies flop in padded pants on to the municipal blue surface. Nude girls do cartwheels. Toddlers swash through the circle of the pool on scooters. A lip smashed on cement is spectacularly bloody and attracts a small crowd. Boys fire dotted arcs of white beads into the air from water guns. Knots of girls screaming and splashing steal the centre of the pool, 30 cm deep at most. Every type of social interaction – trade, fights, sex, feeding, friendship – is being modelled, copied or tried in embryo for the first time. Each day is the creation of the known world over again.

Ev is a negotiator. He navigates the scene. Assessing it for entry points, he is alert for ways to fulfil his desires and he works with the head not the body. Today he ignores the water, but in deep concentration begins with one red lorry. An hour later he has seven vehicles of various types, and a group of toddlers around him, playing on the drain cover closest to the pool.

In an undertow of anxiety that is familiar, I will him to be like the others, or like certain of the others, the young who lord it in the middle of the pool and dare each other on. These are the unequivocal children. About them there is no doubt. I am willing Ev to be more physical, to squeal and jump and act like a child, or at least to get wet. It is stupid. I was never like that. Nor was Tom. Ev wears his red and blue trunks. His sunhat is pushed back on his head. I watch him at his self-made parliament, cajoling, engaging, issuing statements and rounding up fresh players, and my anxiety ebbs away. I keep my distance. Ten minutes becomes fifteen becomes thirty. Finally we leave as the sun is cooling and clouds make a pink line over the houses. He finishes with a swift valediction, a circuit of the water on his scooter. He could pass for any child. *That was a good play*, he says to one of the other boys.

2.7

When the resurrection comes to Herne Hill it will not be as imagined by Stanley Spencer. No. It will be the resurrection as painted by Luca Signorelli in 1500 on the wall of the cathedral at Orvieto, where the immaculate dead lift themselves by their own force, pulling their pristine bodies miraculously out of the smooth, grey piazza. The local council have newly paved the area, taming the junction and doing away with the road to make it continuous with the pavement. They have cleared the way for small armies of café tables to do everlasting battle.

Today I hear the beat of death in all things. I hear it in Brixton, in Stockwell, in Herne Hill, in the streets around the park and off the High Street. It does the thing it has always done; acts as counter and beater and engine, driving blood around my body and to my eyes so that I can see the world before me and all the people in the world afresh. It is in my ears: pumping the blood around the bodies of all the separate people as they move into view going forwards and backwards and always separately to the shops and home and out again to pick up a paper, milk, something they have forgotten, and back again to be with their families at the final hour. 26, 27, 28, 29 ... All is mundane and all is exalted. 81, 82, 83, 84 ...

When I look at Ev, only he eludes this death song. I know why. It is because I cannot see him clearly in the way I cannot see the small of my own back. It is my central pivot but I never get to look at it straight on. Once, Ev was in there himself, pressing against the curve of my spine, fossicking round the vertebrae as he flexed and spun and readied himself in his egg of fluid. *Now*, he was thinking. *Now, it is near*.

Ev's ever-present consciousness and his great unfurling slides of patter run alongside me from about hip level. *My mum made me an omelette and the omelette was tasty it was eggy and so I had an eat. It was a green omelette that my mum made. It was tasty and eggy. I wanted it in triangles. Ham is my best friend. Mum, look! The sky looks like milk! If a cow went on its back its milk would go up into the air*.

This is nothing new or special. This is a child learning to talk, but it is our world he is describing and my ears ping to his voice. Our world is not secure. I strain and bend my body to catch his every utterance and hear us reflected back and back. Mothers do this but here there is more at stake. I spy on him. What does he understand of our situation? I must find out.

In the other room he is explaining us carefully to a friend, paraphrasing and adding to what I had given him earlier. *My dad is a bit stiff and sometimes my mum has to give him a hand. I can't give him a hand because I'm too small.* The friend cuts him off with a question about nursery even though he is uninterested in the answer. No. This is wrong. I will not have it. Ev needs to speak, to repeat. All will be worked out in words. Others need to hear what the boy knows from his own mouth about his own life and his father's dying though they might rather die themselves than hear it or be shrivelled and struck dumb. Embarrassment has supernatural strength.

Ev's hair seen from above is a thick whorl, a dynamo centred on the crown of his head. The cut is growing out Plantagenet and after a long day's play it is stiff with sweat and frizzy with stored energy. Women have twice stopped me in the street to tell me they would pay good money for highlights like that. Its colours are impossible. Alphabetically and incompletely, they are: amber, bronze, butter, citrus, copper, cream, flax, gold, hay, lion, mustard, orange, peach, pink-milk, saffron, straw, tawny, tea and umber. In certain lights it looks green with a chartreuse glaze. I have a yellow leather coat, now too flayed to wear. This coat has the same violent characteristic of yellow-greenness, particularly under neon, as Ev's hair.

We go to a children's party. It is for twin boys: white-faced, red-haired and three years old. In a sensible twist, the hostess has opted out of organisation, structured games and party bags. The house is large, pleasantly dirty and packed with tinies. It is like a set for a Fellini film, an orgy of carpet-level groping, fondling and treading. Each room is primed with babies and toddlers all under a metre. Sometimes three, four deep, they line the stairs and bob around the hall. I count them. There must be more than thirty. There is no floor space to run or pick up any speed so they don't hurt themselves but manoeuvre quite well from room to room like snooker balls, rolling and hitting against padding. Toys spark brief clusters of interest as they settle, skirmish and retreat. All play is in parallel. Busily, constantly, they are shitting themselves and the living room smells of poo on a rolling boil as one child after another is picked from the mass, sniffed and removed. Many mothers are present but as if in a different film. No voices are raised. There are very few tears. It is strangely subdued. The sheer volume of children has the absorbing effect of mattresses stacked against walls. By touch and by feel they soak each other up in empathy. Ev is absorbed and when it is time to go home he is quiet as if deep in thought.

2.8

So. As happens, the future eats the present without sentiment and with straightforward hunger. We are in a position to know. Tom is speaking to me less. We agree. In the automatic formulation of speech, the consciousness that flies out in straight parallel with the word is under strain. Attention and great effort of thought are required and even that may be not enough. The strain fluctuates but at root now it is permanent.

The way his intellect is made manifest through language is being destroyed. Great chunks of speech are collapsing. Holes are appearing. Avenues crumble and sudden roadblocks halt the journey from one part of consciousness to the other. He strings words together like ropes across voids. He is a master improviser, an artist of the swing from thought to word. *Optimism, content, publication*, *orchestra*, *ladder*. Yesterday those words were lost and could not be summoned up or spoken. He got them back today through trial and care but will they be lost again? He never panics. What would it be like if he did? Strategically our lives depend on this aspect of his character. And what happens when those words are lost entirely? No optimism, no content, no publication, no orchestra, no ladder.

His vocabulary is filleted. The lapses may be temporary. After a time he can track them down but they are no longer to hand. As I write – *no longer to hand* – the words are to hand. I know what they are. I know what they mean without thinking about them. I know what order they go in and how to spell them. I know that I can use the phrase *to hand* without referring literally to my own hand. This is no longer his experience. Spelling goes awry or syllables get switched or a likely sound is substituted. The complexity of the problem is so intricate as to be scarcely graspable: sometimes minuscule, like drop-out in a piece of digital music, or then surreal, like the wholesale cut and paste of a message spoken in tongues, at which we all stand astonished, including him. It is a traffic jam inching by degrees. When it becomes chronic, everything stalls. What does *work* mean? What is *of course*? He knows what work means and how to do it. But how do you spell it? In the last two weeks, spelling is gaining as a significant problem. Along the top of his computer I put a strip of masking tape and write in red pen: *a b c d e f g h i j k l m n o p q r s t u v w x y z*. I point out the letters. It works, sort of, for a bit.

We are having lunch in the café in the park and as we eat he relates a conversation he had yesterday with Mark. He had said to him, *Talking used to be such fun*. When I hear this I lower my face on to the white disc of my plate and rest my forehead on its surface. It is a comedy gesture, a side step. I cannot risk a straight one. If I did I would collapse like a puppet in spasm, my joints and connectors violated. No one would be able to put me back together.

Talking used to be such fun. We met in conversation at a party. I'd been in London for only a year after leaving Holland. I had ditched my old happy life with some discontents in search of a new happy one with more structure – if being an artist could be said to have structure – and I was without much firmly established in the way of networks, money or sense of place. I had a horrible studio in King's Cross, a part-time job and an idea about what I wanted to do. With no optimism for the party I had come north on my bike in a spirit, not so much of hedonism but puritanism – much closer to my heart – thinking that socialising in this period of mild drift would be better for me than sitting in my bedsit. The bedsit was often reason enough to propel me out into the night and I was still new enough to be thrilled at cycling across the city in the dark.

I didn't know many there, the hostess, one other and a couple of faces. But I could see that the company was most interesting around him. Tom was drinking happily with a long start on me and not worried about the road home as he lived opposite. What our content was I'm not sure, but the other talkers, a woman and another man, receded. The surface of the table was dotted with foil tops from wine bottles, corks, cigarettes, bits of snacks, spoons, ring-pulls, orange peel, and as we talked his hands were always fiddling with this or that detritus: underscoring a point, rolling a cigarette, pushing things around, orchestrating the surface in front of him like a map or a table-top battle, not really looking at me too much but concentrating on what we were saying. So we began in words. The next day, at twelve o'clock, he called me.

In the space of the last month, words and meanings have been presenting themselves above the surface of the still pool of our existence as if the water that has been evaporating all along had suddenly reached a point where it was noticeable. We are being laid bare. Our waters are receding. Faint white rings of past levels line the walls.

Wordlessness is a symptom of the object-tumour-thing but hand in hand with it is a symptom of its host. Through the last eighteen months he has been producing regularly each week two pieces, 1,500 words and 1,000 words approximately. This is the minimum. Sometimes there is much more. These articles involve going out in the world, looking at artwork, exhibitions, thinking about them and making sense of them. His pieces remain lucid, original and to the point. Funny. His style, always telegraphic – *Why do you make such short sentences?* I used to say – is now more so. He is in danger of self-parody: full stops, commas, dashes and truncations flash and dot all over the text. Here everything flows like language. The work is coherent. It sites itself in the world of legibility and insight. Its aim is to communicate clear things wonderfully well. You can read them. No one would ever know.

These communications are done later and later at night. They take double, near triple the time to write and consume more energy to compose than we can quantify. What does the brain do when it can't reach the phrase *of course*? Where does it go to look for substitutes? Tom was always canny. He waits and he thinks and he waits some more. He does not give up. We are still in the café, my face remains in the plate when he says slowly, *The getting of things exactly right with words, refined and compacted, is my job of many years standing. It is my pride*. The plate holds my cheek and frames the dead weight of my head. It is cool. My eyes are shut. I do not see him, or the café, or the square.

In desperation Ev and I go to the Diana Memorial Playground. He is in my sights.

C'mon. Play, he says, turning to look at me. *Play*.

I'm sad.

You can be sad and still play.

Is the world of the happy different from that of the unhappy? Both states are true and present, both polarities alive in the same moment, cognisant of each other and coexisting. They map exactly. Within the margins that have been given to us, everything is contained, stuck tight against its opposite in full measure, and the friction between them is what makes the life. You cannot help but notice this. If we were to lose this demarcation, if, say, Dr B phoned today to say *It has all been a clinical error*, the friction would vanish. It is total, yet weak as surface tension on a drop of water. There would be no way to mentally attain it or to think yourself back into this state. You cannot pretend to live like this. But it makes the old ways seem intolerable, dependent as they are on pretence.

Trailing Ev as he tacks through the sand, I light up to watch him and I despair as I think of Tom not having this experience now and Ev not having the experience of him to come. It's the same world in the same moment of the world. Dying atoms are contiguous with living atoms but their mass is much heavier, of a weight beyond what I ever thought possible. Ev chases bubbles from a machine shaped like a gun. *Look, Mum, stars, millions of stars!*

2.9

9 July 2010

Dear Friends

It's been three months since Tom's operation. After the latest scan, it appears that the subsequent chemo treatment is not working. Another form of chemo is now being tried out, as of this Monday. This one – PCV – is regarded as being generally more toxic. We don't know how he will react to this. We are anxious.

Tom continues to work well but more slowly. The tumour has always been in the area of speech and language functions, and small changes can have large impact. Though still physically fit, everything becomes much more difficult. We are very tired, except Ev.

This chemo is scheduled to go on for ages and we will need some help in the coming weeks and months. Please let us know if you have some nice ideas, food is always good, as is childcare, normality, outings and conversation. Just staying in touch at this time is really important to us. Forgive us if we don't immediately get back to you, but do continue to write, phone, text, email, invite and visit us.

Thanks as ever for your support. We look forward very much to seeing you.

With love

The cornfield pans out low in front of me. It is a basic landscape scene. The horizon holds the field flat in its dish. Silhouettes of deer break the skyline and telephone wires mark out the sky in radiating segments. To the right is a one-track road and on the other side are woods and a bridleway. Ahead is all farmland. There is no wildness and the land carries everywhere the print of maintenance and marks of use, yet encroachment feels not so far off, as if left to itself the land would slip back in a short year: paths covered with brambles, fields threaded with weeds. Our friends' house is the middle one in a row of three cottages built around each other and set at odds to a road running between one hamlet and the next. Roses loop about the brick. We are back in the place where it all started.

That was nearly two years ago. In the middle of the night, I had been woken by Tom having a violent fit and in its aftermath the green and yellow hard body of the ambulance taking him away was like a tropical insect vanishing into darkness as if it had never been there, as if Tom was not in it. The night folded in like black dough behind. Ev and I followed in the car with the first response nurse. Her steady neutral chatter – cut-backs to the emergency system, the role of the first response team – was enough to carry the silence yet give me an entry should I want to talk. *Am I on holiday? What a beautiful child. What work do I do?* I remember Ev's sleeping face glowing as we drove out of the woods and into the town, by car-light, then street-light, then day-light; red, white, yellow, orange, blue.

All the next day we hung around the dead end hospital. Ev was in animal mode, breastfeeding madly, a hot weight hanging on my neck. I thought my milk should have turned but it remained sweet. It was a bank holiday and the hospital was not shut down but one level up from that; wholly downgraded. All day I watched as Tom slept and woke and slept and on each waking became more fluent and more himself. I saw his mind going to work. It was a visible act of summoning, consciousness forming itself into a shape. And then when he asked for his laptop, I saw too his writing creeping out like a file of ants as he typed all the wrong words.

But over the day it got better and better, language, writing, better and better. I felt oddly like we had had luck, as if some giant, mysterious thing had been avoided, though I had no evidence for this. The doctors wondered if it had been a minor stroke. A CAT scan gave no clear conclusion. When there was nothing more to be learned, Ev and me went back to the house to wait. The evening had turned so pale and gold it was near transparent and after I put Ev to bed, I stood for a long time looking towards the far edge of the cornfield until just as the sky blooded from rose to red, my phone rang. It was Tom: back and fully present in his own voice, cheering and comforting me.

How do we recognise another person? At its most basic, by shape, by colour, by outline, by dark and light, by smell. Or by nuances of tone, by the way the face looks in repose, the cadences of the voice, full of small interior knowledge, the way they hold their mouth while listening, or the way their gaze holds yours. By what their eyes say when they are not speaking.

That day had ended in the same warm darkness. Finally he was allowed to leave and he came home very late, exactly as himself, but glittering, talking fast and full, full of joy, exhausted and energised and moving lightly on the balls of his feet. His eyes seemed newly membraned. Something had happened. An event.

We have not set foot in the cottage since then and this can't be explained in terms of superstition. We are not inclined to that. It's more that a faint audio wave, a clang of hurt, attaches to it like a far-off bell. Now we have four days to spend here and the schema we make is for sleep, beach walks and long evenings. We are a high risk, it is acknowledged. Anything may happen to us at any time. Time expands in chaotic, unforeseen ways. We seem to have a lot of it at our disposal although of course in terms of numbered days and years we have less. These days are no exception.

Reprise. Tom is doing the early shift, to let me lie in, when he has a serious seizure. For the second time we call an ambulance. He comes round with five of us standing over him like giants. The ceiling is too low to accommodate an emergency: the tall paramedics and their equipment crowd again under the beams of the cottage. We eye him carefully. He eyes us back. *Yes. OK. Good*. He is returning.

Ever so slowly we inch back on to the barely functioning platform that is our life. Our friends are stoic, but ashen. Fit witnessing is a hard business. My heart flutters. Maybe it is I who will die.

Cancer scarcely allows you time to look at it, let alone get used to it. Tom's is a high-speed disease with full, motorway pile-up repercussions. It does not pause to allow you to admire the view from anywhere. How many times do I think, *Now we are really in trouble*. Well, on this page I say it again. Now, we are really in trouble. And this time I mean it more than all the previous times. But there will surely be another time when I will mean it more still and this time will seem as nothing. This time will seem manageable or benign in retrospect. We may look back on it and laugh, though I suspect we will not find quite the right vantage point to do that.

Back at home I am ranting. We need another strategy. This one isn't working. Maintaining the thinnest facade of a functioning family that tries to act as others do – plan ahead, drive somewhere, go on holiday, relax – is beyond us. We are smashed. Insecurity jams the gears on every action. Each time we are toppled. I feel a fool over and over again for trying. Easier please to abandon the pretence. Easier surely, to stop. Stop and not try.

In the middle of my outburst Tom interrupts me. *I am frightened.* What? I have not heard this before. He is my balance, my bar, the surface on which I put my feet, the edge I trace my hands around so I can see where I am going even in the dark. *I am frightened*, he says. He is right to be so. I repeat and repeat. *I am here. We are here. I am here. We are home.*

Ev goes to the cousins for the weekend, where he is absorbed into a five-headed child-organism. He will make a pair with the youngest and play with the train track or in the garden, with trucks, earth and dirt. We have two days when we can sleep in, to nine, ten, twelve and beyond, perhaps to nine again.

When he comes home he tries out his new phrase. *I'm sad about Dad.* This is Ev's gambit. *Why is he ill?* He asks, *Is it because he has flootens?* He roars with laughter.

2.10

We almost miss it. The doors are closing. We throw ourselves on to seats opposite each other on the Tube. Around us the carriage is assembling at the last minute ready to move off. People eat, read the papers, fuss with bags and scuff their feet. They shift and re-settle. No one notices us.

Tom looks across at me, placed fresh in front for his inspection. He sees how I have landed, occupying one seat and part of the neighbouring one in a sideways slouch, my legs tucked wilfully into themselves. He sees my coat with the black collar sticking up lopsided, buttons undone. The threads in the weave of the coat look dark, near black, but are really green. He bought it for me in Paris and we didn't notice the refinement until I got it home. My hair is thick and blunt, unbrushed. I know this because I am reflected in the window behind him.

Through familiarity my face must be hard to see. That's what I find with his. If you were to meet him, you would not think that such a lot was going on. He has a dark brown beard, flecked with white. A moustache balances out the beard that would look Amish or insane without it. Thick bushy eyebrows gone into old man hair sit above very blue eyes. When we met it was the eyes that were the main draw. He looks well for a man on toxins. His weight is too high but his skin is healthy and his hair chemo-curly. More strangely, I look well. I am in a phase – there are only ever phases in sequenced strings – where stress causes me to produce handsome chemicals like expensive scent. It is a natural collagen. I have fuller, thicker hair and my legs are browning from afternoons at the paddling pool with Ev.

I cannot describe myself in words. My face is thinner. I have lost weight of course. Dark crescents of bruised skin start in the corner of my eyes and curve under the bottom lid. I have had these for as long as I can remember but now they are heraldic. Sleep deprivation, from Ev's early waking and Tom's narcotic disorders, is at an all-time high. I pay both more and less attention to myself. Less attention to how I feel, as in *my own needs,* as they are sometimes called. These are beyond analysis. But I pay a bit more attention to how I look, as if attending to the surface will hold it all temporarily together or at least give me that valuable ounce more traction and spring, like a runner trying out a new shoe to gain a couple of seconds over the track.

We exist as much as the other bodies in the carriage exist. No one would know any different. It is a caprice, a slight. Death's jest. We appear to be willed creatures, like them on the way to somewhere, heads down and busy with all our choices: where to live, what to eat, how to dress, who to love, what to think, what to desire. We are on our way to see the neurologist. *This is mad*, Tom says. I nod. Mute.

2.11

My job is threefold.

1. Not to let Tom be destroyed before his death but to help him live it fully in his own way with all his power.
2. Not to let Ev be destroyed by Tom's death but to help him live it fully in his own way with all his power.
3. Not to let myself be destroyed. See 1 and 2.

That's it.

I am an over-achiever. I will do anything and everything and all. Why am I so competitive? Must I do even this thing well? This is a time of sureness. Even now we are happy. Yet if I still cannot call myself unhappy what does that mean? That I am enjoying myself? Is it so ingrained in me that to live is to be happy that I must spin the story of a death, a blinding, catastrophic death in the middle of my life, if not to my advantage – beyond me – then not precisely to my disadvantage? The stakes are stratospheric. My thoughts are ragged as pre-formed clouds. The air is so thin it lightens my head. To die is the whole of the work. Yet to survive is identical with it. Survival means survival for all of us, in such diverse ways as we may.

The project is not to go down. It is all or none. One down. All down. Tom, being dead, will survive for us. His memory, his words and his work spreading outwards will shade the things we have and colour the things we will have in the future. For Ev and me, surviving means not being annihilated by his absence. Not being destroyed by the manner of it. There is nothing here to be angry about. It is fantastical. It is all to play for.

The template of self-image I adhere to is that of a happy person. Is this different from being happy? I have no idea. Before the crisis, the bad sank down somewhere I couldn't reach or was too lazy to get to, and the good floated up as flotsam near the surface. I was usually near the surface too, sometimes impressively active and sometimes just bobbing and lolling, lolling and rolling, the one a front for the other. *Bad* and *Good* are weakened words now, blanched of force. Language is failing me too.

Optimism is an under-researched attribute. Where's the science? Where's the research? What do our brother creatures – the owls, crabs, bonobos – think about the bright side? What do optimists do under pressure? Do they continue to seek out slivers of silver the size of fingernails in the crushed, smashed and folded lining of the earth? Optimism doesn't seem to be something you can just adopt. Equally, I can't be rid of it, even in mid-fall. It can seem so much the wrong response, inappropriate, like an embarrassing social tic. I don't mean I have optimism about our outcome. I know the outcome. I don't even mean that I think it will be easy. We may be spared in some way, we may, we may not. And yet ... I know us.

I am a blessings counter. I am and always was. My family gifted me balance and ballast. By upbringing and temperament it was just one of those things that came with me. I link it to the most rudimentary physical sense of being-in-the-world: sun on skin, smell, particular light, that sort of stuff, and that in turn connects to the articulation of the stretch between being an individual – myself – and non-individuated matter. I have always been able to think of myself as matter: one and many, all-solipsist and nothing at all. Not anything.

As a teen I was a megalomaniac and part-time visionary. We lived for a while in a small Scottish town and often I would stand after school on the hill behind our house, *The Vertish*, it was called, and look down at the town without being in any way attentive to its detail – slate roofs, the ragged line of lights climbing the hill, the dark cut of the river – I knew all that. But more I was feeling its topography, its volume and weight, rills and falls. I could see how the place inhabited three dimensions on the land and how the shape of the land fixed it under the blackening sky. I could see the things that had been built and the things that couldn't be described exactly as made but more had adjusted themselves over time to what was there already: growths, outcrops, promontories. And from my vantage I could view the place, me the viewer, and everything in it from all angles at once: from my side of the valley and the other, from above, from the neck of the town, down its flank and from its pit.

It would be years before I saw a 3D simulation. This was something of the same experience though fundamentally different in that it wasn't a constructed reality, one that had to be imagined piece by piece to be achieved, but a purely *felt* sight. I understood it without effort or strain. I could do this because all the matter in the visual field, myself included, was undifferentiated, part of the same stuff. To see was to be. Viewed like this, the visual, even when applied to a small Scottish border town as remote, hermetic and unpromising as this one, was a complex, wild and extravagant place. Spatial sense was magic sense. Still is. As I said, I was a megalomaniac but I didn't really know the word.

But I speak too soon. The question of happiness is previous. Tom is still here. We cannot escape being here until we do and we will not comprehend not being here when we are not. It is endemic. Back then on the hill, my imagination was not constrained. Now I am dumb as to what happens after.

Tom is in the bedroom. He is finding a book for me. Opening it to mark a poem. It is one of many that he once knew by heart and cannot now speak: Empson, Larkin, Beddoes, Heaney, Hill. He knows where everything is on the shelf. He cannot read books exactly but he knows them. He has wit and capacity to look them up and he does it with purpose and for me.

Here he is now at the fridge, scanning it for something to eat. There's a casual intelligence in what he does: seeks out old lettuce to throw away, pushes back the eggs, shuffles the milk, makes a bit of space, hunts down snacks. And outside, I see only his back this time as he walks away from me with Eric, their heads bent together in talk. He can still arrange words like blocks to create a connection. A word is a thing in the head. Well this one here is a knife. This one a sock tucked in on itself. This is the book you were looking for. This is the word *home*. With these he can build a new thing to be said and responded to.

Maybe all that can be spoken by me at this time is not about happiness or unhappiness, or optimism or competition, but just that we are all still here. To be still here is all there is. This page marks our presence. In the light of that fact either I do not despair or I suppress despair, I cannot tell which. Plenty of time to work that out later.

2.12

In Wrocław the air was animal, vegetable and mineral, not like any air I had ever breathed. It was heavily polluted. The colours of a winter evening were coal and smoke and iron and fire. Darkness drew a soft hood over the head. On Christmas Eve, live carp swam out their last hours in baths set in the street in preparation for the evening feast. The next day the Ceauçescus were butchered on my small black and white television. And on the last day of 1989 I went to Berlin along with everyone else for the great party following the destruction of the wall.

I lived in Wrocław for nine months on a scholarship at the Art School and learned Polish fast. My father speaks many languages and I am good at that sort of thing so it was easy but the speed of it was considered on the ground as some kind of local phenomenon. Unlike my father, my language included many swear words merrily acquired in a scattershot way without benefit of context or etiquette. What was passable for a man to say was not in order for a lady. Swearing on all the intimacies of the body is mainstream Polish man-talk. One day my friend Marek, himself a handy swearer, had had enough. He rebuked me in a whisper, *Jak brzidki mówisz – How dirty you talk*. I cleaned up.

In bed at night I think of other languages. Polish, Dutch from Amsterdam, bad Italian from Rome. One can be simply other by taking on alternative structures and sounds. You can learn to float in water. You can learn buoyancy through language: liberation from syntax and meaning. In Poland at that time inflation was rocketing each day and necessity was the driver as I haggled over tomatoes or tried to buy wet chunks of *biały ser.* I had to find words to stop the dinner lady in the canteen putting gravy on my potatoes. Why I was a vegetarian in Poland I can't remember. But those were local skirmishes. I could trade on novelty and be a more forward version of myself. I didn't wait to learn a word before trying it but tried it on first hearing and if it didn't work, well, there was no loss. Tomorrow I would try again to buy tomatoes and today onions on black bread with salt would do.

Words as guesswork, play, as joint enterprise, as joke, as game. This is all useful to me now.

What else is there apart from language? Let me list: music, touch, the great inter-cosmos of the eyes, running and jumping, sex, cooking, friendship, eating. There must be other things but I have come to a stop. It's a short list. We will devise another language and in it we will talk.

We discuss strategies. One is to verbally go for broke. Tom could learn to accept a percentage of nonsense in the interests of volubility in a sort of trade, not waiting to get things right but crashing in, usurping the speech habits of a lifetime. He has noticed that he can sometimes get more done by taking a jump at language, not going so much for style. It is the automatic bits that are the problem. It might have diminishing returns but it is a way. This will be hard for him. It is a Blurters' manifesto. To be truly comprehensible, everything he says has to be thought out first. He must think very hard before he speaks. We, who do not think before we speak, speak, and the thought is there, full-spake, articulate. It sits like a jelly on a plate before us. This morning Ev is making nonsense noises in our bed. *Does Dad need pills because he gets his words muddled? Yes. Is that you trying to muddle your words, Ev? No. I am making bubble noises.*

The three-month span is up again and it is time for the oncologist. We go in the mood of holding steady, hoping nothing, fearing nothing, positioned in each other's company and moving through the stages that tend to fall before appointments: the number three bus, walking, bloods, weighing, waiting, with a kind of cool, a knowledge that whatever we felt would not change the outcome and therefore we could feel just as we chose, steady, alive and together.

The outcome is bad. (Did I know this in advance? Again that weird trick: knowledge falls on to ground that seems ready prepared though you never remember doing it.) The scan is hard to decipher in a way that doesn't look good. OK. What do we do now? Second opinion. Talk to the surgeon, look at other chemo options, all of them more retro. In the beginning our drugs were state of the art. We move backwards in time and opportunity and if a drug were so good, we would have been there already. Surgery: three surgeries, can that even be an option? It is mentioned. The last one scraped a fresh hole in Tom's head and altered mine profoundly. If I were a tree you would find traces of that date, 13 April 2010, in my wood. It would register as a disturbance in my rings, a disruption, a check in growth, a wound.

After the oncologist I pick up Ev from nursery. I am not making much headway with other parents. This is understandable. I don't have the mental reach, the open arms. A group of parents from the nursery are aware of what is going on with us and that is some relief. But the nursery itself is not a relief. It is a modern building, bright, generous and well designed with curved walls in sunflower yellow. Blue lino, eco displays and plastic furniture all converge in an environment dedicated to the future. I cannot stand it. The future will not relent.

Children are the raw, soft part of us and because of Ev I am at my most vulnerable here. Our family trauma is a monster. I cannot casually let it out near the sandpit and the dressing-up box. The adults you meet here are contingent. All interactions are distracted and conducted over the heads of the young. This is not an environment for the formal presentation of pain. There is no way to do it that protects me and there is never a right time. When I try, the result is demolition. Tears stop my mouth before I can continue. I leave as fast as I can and feel the impact in fatigue for days.

I do not need new friends to support me. I have enough. But I have to keep coming here and unless I am truthful, the fiction is created that I am just like them and that Ev is just like their children. Keeping up this fiction is so tiring. But then the other way, to speak the truth when they ask lightly, *Oh, how are you?* I seek the way of least struggle and lightest pain. The nursery staff do the only thing they can. They are wildly generous in their attention and care of Ev.

Sometimes what I want to explain to Ev is this:

Look, I can be rougher than I should be with a three-year-old whose father is dying. This is because the shape of the person that you see here is held in place by pressure and will and by contingencies of illness or wellness like whether your father can talk to me or not today.

What I feel as I watch you a living/living being and he a dying/living being seems supernatural. I don't know why I am not mad, or blind. But I am not. Still, we have this life and we float about in it and many things continue to happen to us for very good and very ill. I am not dissolved. I do not moan or despair. I do not panic. But I am über-naturally tired. The edges of my vision are distorted. The fibre of my muscles is weak. My tongue lacks spring. My hands do not rest. Pressure can cause me to lose my shape under tension and when this happens I lose my temper. I regret this. Some obscure, scratchy line will be crossed, a transgression so minor you might not feel the violation. This must be confusing I know. It is textbook bad child-rearing, signals hopelessly mixed. But it happens and there are worse things.

(But then I remember that the worse thing is also happening.)

First – if I am outright wrong and haven't even been provoked, we apologise and kiss. I try to close the gap between flare and kiss, to a hiss, a hiatus. I learned not to sulk or go cold on you a long time ago. My anger is condensed, hot and translucent, not icy or opaque. I never leave you guessing.

Second – if I am sort-of-right to lose my temper and much provoked, we apologise and kiss. You see – the outcome is the same. We end in each other's arms. So, forgive.

Tom says, *He is so bold and you are sometimes so rough with him, yet he always comes straight back*. I think about this for a while. *If I am sometimes rough with him*, I say, *it is through fear of the void.* What if he had no one to say, *Come-and-finish-your-dinner*, or *Get-down-here-right-now* or *It-is-time-to-go-to-bed-I-told-you-twice-already*. How would he feel then? Alone. I cannot bear this. My insistence on sitting down to eat, cleaning teeth or tidying toys is a way of holding on to living as practice, as routine. It is all so volatile with us. We need to hold this stuff in sight.

Then I continue: *And if he comes straight back it shows that he is secure in my love. This is a fact about him that I should not take lightly*. Almost in passing a friend comments that it would be easy to lose your temper with a three-year-old even under normal circumstances, without brain cancer to contend with. Sounds perfectly true. But I realise suddenly that I have no grasp of what normal circumstances might be, and as I leave her I am ever so slightly salved. Anointed. Lighter.

There is violence of course. The mother–child relationship is a testing ground for all permutations of all relationships. Violence comes within its remit. Ev started to hit my face when he was about one year old. Out of affection, boredom or delight, to get a reaction, or my attention, or just to gauge the sound it made, I don't know. It went on for months and like a drip-drip torture it was the crack that wore through. My response time was slowed by pheromones. I just wasn't quick enough to escape his fat paw. He had surprising heft for a baby and always worked at very close range. Putting him to bed while snuggling or stroking his hair was a favourite moment. *Whack*. Or as I hugged him close to my body, savouring the warmth of his torso and feeling his lovely weight, he would rear back to get some distance. *Whack*. On sleep portioned into three-hour blocks I can't swear to my response. I tried retreating, storming out, reasoning with him or just bawling, DON'T HIT MY FACE. Minutes later I would be back in the only place I wanted to be, my face inches from his. *Whack*.

I am there now. Ev is right next to me and together we watch the sunset fade. He wriggles and snuggles, his movements winding down, smaller and softer: slower. He is drifting. His eyelashes, the second thing I registered at birth after the exquisite, fine penwork of his lips, are enormous. They curve graciously over closed eyes: small shadows drawn neatly beneath, the mark of intensive play. This is the end of his last week at little nursery. *Have you had a good week, Ev? Have you enjoyed yourself? Yeh*. He is half-smiling at me. *Yeh*.

What an impossible creature. How remote is early childhood. He is an island boy to our city dwellers. Here is someone so proximate to our lives – 10 cm from my face and breathing calmly – yet untouchable. Can this be so? This has been one of the worst weeks ever, an appalling week, difficult in ways I can't quantify. For Tom, drugged out of shape, it has been peaceful. No sickness, just the limbo of unconsciousness interrupted by eating, waking, not speaking much, bits of work. Yet here we are. It is Friday night. We are at the week's end and Ev, his child, is smiling and relaxed, happy and about to sleep. I believe him. He does not dissimulate. What a wonder. The accelerating forces of Ev's life are a perfect counterweight to the forces accelerating in ours. He can deal with it all and he will. I trust him. He is a true master.

2.13

You should know that I am a slob and I love to loll. I do not wish to have the roles I have: cook, facilitator, interpreter, editor, carer, watcher, driver, calendar keeper, drug administrator, planner, gatekeeper, worrier, conduit, walker, helper, organiser, nag, mother.

We move deeper into the land of the unreal. It all seems silly, childish. A game has gone wrong. The rules are arbitrary. No one can remember them anyway but the results are fatal. There has been black propaganda against him. A decision has been made in secret. Tom is being sent away, reason unknown, discriminated against and told he cannot play with us any more. It is a procedural matter. We have no right of appeal. That fact alone drives us mad. How we love to argue and appeal. It's the whole of our fun. We sit opposite each other on one of our many evenings, he on the collapsing pink sofa now beginning to double as his bed and me on the derelict blue one. We are alive, as alive as you. Yet we are to stop.

It is the first week of August. Andy comes to stay and we go to the Heath, walking very slowly up the hill to the flouncing kites, and take up a position to watch them. Tom sits on the bench, his face turned to the sky, and the rest of us lie on the grass like fallen shapes in a fitful hotness. Ev throws himself on each of us in turn and Andy and I toss him on our upturned feet, roll him down the hill and tickle him till he farts.

But over the following days many things happen. Events collapse into one another and occurrences are set in train with their ends not in sight. It starts with a physical manifestation so at odds with the problems we have come to know – fits or fatigue or dysphasia – that it takes us by surprise. Diarrhoea mixed with bright red, new blood. This is enough to get us into hospital but under our own steam, without many qualms. Like a battered old dualist I reason – this is the body, just blood and shit, this is not the bad brain dealing its next bad hand, it is matter and hospitals deal perfectly well with matter. They must have gallons of it going in and out all the time. So we check ourselves in, not calmly surely, but in charge, texting gaily all the while on the first evening. *All procedures going! xx t*. It will be a respite courtesy of the NHS in a not-so-great part of town but we will both be able to get some sleep. Indeed on the first night it is true. I get seven hours unbroken. I cannot remember feeling like this for so long: like a bell struck or a freshly cleaned and folded towel. But the next day when I visit, Tom is in pain so that's the end of it. No more nights like that. So far we have not had pain, scarcely a pill's worth. Whatever the tumour has been getting up to, it has not hurt.

Food poisoning, the doctors hazard. Andy, just back from Ethiopia, who had cooked us the Berbere fish the night before, is distraught. Ev gets wind of it. *Did Dad eat all the red fish?* Infection is the next guess, so they keep him in isolation. He is in hospital for six days and though the pain, the blood and the shit recede, for six days and nights he stays on his own in a small room like a cell painted cream, turquoise and lilac with a window view aslant over the pure arse of south London: undefined, undignified and stretching to the horizon.

After tests they determine colitis. This is a problem but it can be treated and seems anyway to be easing off of its own accord. Its root is unclear but what is clear is that a brain already stressed by a tumour can collapse very suddenly under pressure of physical illness. The brain is metabolically hungry. Here it is being starved. Tom becomes timid and unsure. In the space of six days he gets confused and his language fails harder. His morale goes lower than I have ever seen. He has the sheer ability and reason to ride high most of the time. He is buoyant. We all cling to this. *A floater*, he calls himself. Yet it is Friday, he is being discharged but we are struggling to convince him. He worries he won't be able to climb the stairs at home or get up from the bed; he whines about getting dressed, about getting into the car. He doesn't want to go. I pretend not to be astonished. I edit my voice to keep the surprise out of it but my heart bangs in my chest. What is this? He is changed.

One phenomenon irritates me beyond sense. He will not look at me. In the little cell he does not meet my eye. His voice is dull and without colour. *I am over here*, I keep saying. *Hello. I am here, look at me!* I wave at him rudely inches from his face. I am belligerent because I am afraid. *Here I am working to spring you from this hospital and the least you can do is look at me.* I tell him he has Stockholm syndrome and the hospital is his captor but he scarcely rises to this drollery. We have to get out of here.

I remind him how much he wants to see Ev. Truly Ev is more than he can cope with right now but our love for our children is supposed to be one of those universal and sustaining stimuli that never fails to work so I throw it in anyway.

The best nurses have the miraculous facility of instant appraisal – praise to their Patron Saint. The nurse Sheila grasps what is going on and she and I make common purpose and work on him together. *Just wait till you feel the air on your face again after all this time. Wait till you get back in your own environment, it will all seem different. Let's get you home to eat some proper food. You can go home and get some work done. All your friends can start to come again.* As we say this, I don't know what she is thinking but I think that we are bluffing. But it comes to pass exactly so. In everything we say, we are right. In the end Tom creeps out of the ward, his face stony, warding me off as a potential foe. But I cannot help noticing that he is in the passenger seat of the car quicker than I can get his bags stowed and turn to help him. This is a sign. I am galvanised. Keeping up a pure tonic of talk like a stream of energising bubbles I drive out and round towards the Elephant and Castle breathing in the air. It is heaven this air. Even as we exit I can feel the man next to me returning, his resurgence following the curve of the roundabout, his body bending softer into the seat as we stream out of the slip road in the direction of home. He winds down the window. *Ah yes,* he says. *Ah yes.*

Just before we leave, Sheila takes me to one side to talk about Tom's new drugs. He came in with two, Epilim and dexamethasone, both self-administered, morning and evening. Now I am handed eight in a green, sealed plastic bag with an instruction chart I know he cannot follow in his present state. I panic. It is wrong to say the word *Fuck* in hospital. Not a sweary house this. The elderly shouty man outside Tom's cell, who we call Falls Risk from the sign written in pen above his bed, says *Fuck* a lot but that is his prerogative. What is it not to cope? Not to cope means to fail. What is that, to fail?

Although there is more to come, of course more and I cannot pretend to be wise about it, I think I have a sense now of what it all is and what it all will be. And what do I think? Everything that can be said has been said before, either in the same or a different way and can be said in other ways again. There is comfort in this. Yet it doesn't go the other way. I can never say about Tom losing his words, *Ah well, it is only words.* There are 88,298 words in this book. But this is nothing. Not even the beginning.

2.14

It is the middle of the day and I have gone to bed. Being tired is the cover but in fact I am plain pissed off, fed up, done in. Our coordinates are bust. That's what I'm thinking. Three points on a graph can generate a conversation. One to two, one to three, two to one, two to three,

three to one, three to two. Three points makes a system of simple complexity, early-stage proliferation. If you were to draw between three points you would get a shape: one edge a base and the other two supporting. Or vice versa. A basic structure. A tent.

Two points go: one to two, two to one, one to two, two to one and back, endlessly, to infinity shuttling back and forth like an echo. It's a recipe for madness. If you were to draw between two points you would get a line. A line is a point moving through space. It has breadth but its main matter is extension. A line is not a shape. A line is not in two dimensions. You could overdraw the line and after a while the paper would tear. A line is weakness. Any way you look at it, it's the same. Yesterday we had an important conversation with Dr B, the oncologist, a catch-up in a month of gathering trouble. These days we know everything before she does and her tests simply confirm our knowledge. It feels natural to us to know. We are illness embodied after all and have been so for a long time.

All this month we have watched the outline and edge of change shape itself before our eyes. We note the demarcation lines of illness and wellness, their borders tingling on alert, glowing green, soft and elastic, looping and curling to draw new phenomena ever within their reach and scope. *This too! Ah yes of course! This too! You didn't think you would be spared this?* Everything has a side effect somewhere else. Drugs layer new problems over old like fresh scabs. Limb weakness, that's because the steroids are too high. Tiredness is down to metformin or chemo. Shaky hands means the Epilim needs adjusting. Swollen feet is diabetes. Shit equals colitis. Speech difficulties, well, the steroids are too low. It is a sinuous disease. What did we talk about with the oncologist yesterday? I had a list. Twelve points. Numbered.

We proceeded methodically down the page of my little book, deviating when the conversation got more interesting or jumped ahead. A landslide of information was marshalled. Things got repeated, noted down, attention paid. We are still reverent to the facts. The force of our attention was fit to crush the facts to dust.

For the first time she brings up the name of the drug Avastin. It was in the headlines only two days ago – did I read it? I read nothing. Words pass my eyes like objects on a conveyor and sometimes they filter from there into my head. My receptors for information have always been sharp. Now they are extrasensory. I am a new type of being. I can smell out what I need and scent it blind. Certainly I do not consciously read. My concentration is too poor to take in information in lines of words massed in blocks with breaks between. That is old-fashioned. I have been honed into modernity these last two years. We both of us are extremely up-to-date and modern and we stand at the forefront and the edge.

Avastin is the next agent that might be employed against Tom's cancer. The word *drug* has disappeared overnight from our vocabulary and has been replaced by the more progressive *agent*. Drug bad. Agent good. It is a long shot. Licensed in America, but not here, Avastin needs special dispensation from the Primary Care Trust and Dr B will draft a letter outlining his case. Now I remember the headline. I read it over someone's shoulder on the Tube. Avastin costs £21,000 per course of treatment.

2.15

So. Everyone is going round like tourists. It is the last week in August: a perfect pocket of hell. Friends and professionals are all out of reach while we three are on something like a luge: Olympic, gigantic, at the top end of the sport. Unfortunately we are amateurs.

August from its first to its last day has been like this, a designated disaster zone, dates crossed out on the calendar like grazes or scars and dotted with emergency notes scribbled in pen. In the giant City State of the hospital, new doctors take up their posts in early August and the convulsion of their arrival continues until the end of the month when gone-away staff return from the beaches and rocks of France and Croatia to face the great wave of September's fresh sick and maimed. Emails go unanswered, messages do not get passed on, dates for procedures come and go, Post-it notes go missing and questions float wistfully in the air. Meanwhile we, outside the institution, outside of everything, are well under way on our own steam. We howl along, all three of us together, with knocks and shocks and sudden up-speedings round curves skewed tight enough to spill us right out, and our bones and skin are broken and torn but there is always more bones and skin to be mangled. Like a miraculous Catholic bloody endurance sport, there is always more. In the space of three weeks, between us we have had hospital stays, fits, diarrhoea, speech loss, tonsillitis, swollen feet, mobility loss, demoralisation, ambulances, glue ear and holidays – everything happens always and forever, on holiday. But we are not tourists. We travel tightly baggaged with our lives. There is nothing left at home.

There is a mill in Norfolk. This is where we are going. It is a monopod with no sails, its circular foot planted like a surveyor on the land looking in the direction of the sea. This is a holiday with other families squeezed on to the end of a summer of going nowhere. I don't tell Ev what we are doing until we get here because I am unsure that we can achieve anything we set out to do and don't want to disappoint him in whatever he thinks holiday means.

In seven floors ascending the mill holds its ground for miles. At the top are the innards of its machinery, a giant grindstone smoothed with pigeon shit and dust. Going down, the next habitable floor has iron beds for lying on stiff as dead knights and windows with makeshift curtains, their colours leached by the sun over decades. Each floor as you descend has marginally more comfort. The first is relatively opulent: radiators, framed watercolours, bedside lamps, rugs and gigantic dark wooden furniture. The first floor is where most people stay and children mainly venture higher to sleep if they can goad each other into bravery against the dark, citing ghosts and cobwebs. There are blankets and crockery enough for a small field hospital. If ever a war came, it would be a good place to be. Most of the living is done on the ground floor in a large circular room like a compendium of vintage domesticity, packed with sofas, games, harmonium, tables, cushions, cards, piano and books.

The morning after we arrive Tom has a major seizure. Danuta is the doctor we fetch up with at the local hospital and I do not warm to her. She is wearing black, and her sallow, circular face, sloping torso and round hips make three spheres, like a bitter snowman. Throughout our discussion she keeps her arms folded against me. Clearly she would rather be elsewhere. It is 9 p.m., a Monday night, and over the day he has got palpably better. Martha is with me and we are arguing that Tom needs to be released from this place because anything they might do can wait until he gets back to London to reconnect with the vast army of professionals who know a great deal about him already.

It is a long discussion and I never quite work out what Dr Snowman's point is, though she is adamant about it. No, he must stay: it is dangerous, another fit is possible, something new, or maybe not new has been seen on the CAT scan, further observation is needed. As the wife, I am at a disadvantage. Dr Snowman has the authority of the medical profession. We are stuck.

The hospital is chaotic. A Polish man in paper underpants in the next bed shouts all through our discussion, falls several times to the floor and begins to finger his way playfully into our bay, clawing at the curtain and swearing the while. My knowledge of Polish curses is extensive, so I can interpret this for Martha. Dr Snowman can do it herself. She is undermined and getting rattled. She calls repeatedly for the staff nurse when it looks like the Pole may be about to spring an entry on to Tom's bed. To remain here is dangerous. Escape is our best action.

It's so noisy in here my brain is pulped and I understand her less and less. Tom, still recovering, cannot follow her argument at all. He looks suddenly very vulnerable. Dr Snowman is failing to outline the risks coherently enough that we can make a choice and I figure this probably signals her argument is running into the ground. Finally I say, *Enough. We are leaving.* We sign ourselves out on a green form acknowledging that we and we alone bear all the risks that follow by discharging ourselves. As we wait in the corridor I see that the women's bay is a model of decorum while in the men's the apes are running wild.

Staff Nurse Curtis has heard the whole of our negotiations over the swearing of the Pole. *I think you are doing the right thing,* she says. This intelligent piece of kindness, freely given, is an act of love. We look at her. Suddenly, as if wound up and released, she sets off running very fast down the empty corridor in search of a wheelchair to speed us on. In amazement we watch her back disappearing round the corner.

But back at the mill directly on our return, small fits are coming in waves. His drugs are not in control. These are verbal tremors from which he extricates himself over several minutes, his sentences slowly building back into coherence in a reverse countdown. I record this process on the phone to the emergency services lady as we wait to see which way it will go. It is a tense moment, one of the worst. It is nearly midnight. The situation unfolds in the circular room to the accompaniment of my commentary on the phone and as they listen the children melt away, uncurling from sofas and books with discreet backward glances. Though I recognise this from minor incidents in my childhood – the finely balanced tension between see or flee, embarrassment, shock at adults up-ended, pity – I wish it were not so. I wish they would stay and see it for what it is. What do they say to each other in the bedrooms upstairs? Perhaps nothing, too awful to speak of, or whispered explanations tried out for the younger ones. No matter.

I am losing you.

Yes, I know.

The next day we are fine. This is how it goes. I am in the sea. Tom sleeps in the sun on the beach. Ev plays nearby. The air is a hair-dryer on its lowest setting, blowing a warm and happy storybook wind. The sea at low tide is the same temperature as the air but of a brown texture thick with sand. Warmth dries us in seconds and makes a strange fusion with the water that in contrast seems barely wet. I swim with Martha and Mo and our three heads poke above the water. Suddenly a fourth person appears, a child, quite near. I am surprised, where did he come from so suddenly? He's a funny-looking boy in a tight grey and black cap. I catch his profile and recognise him. A seal. He holds his neck so human, shoulders sloping under the waves as he looks at us, that I laugh aloud. His doggy snout and whiskers are up for play and he heads towards Martha, black eyes gleaming. It is exhilarating to swim the four of us together. We were four people connected in consciousness, when one of us was unmasked as an impersonator. The seal disappears. He can out-swim us all freely and wildly; we check the waters around our legs for his presence.

2.16

On one given day this is what happens. Today the sum of people arriving is greater than usual. Some days there may be almost nobody, although that hasn't happened for a while, but today is not untypical in the unfolding of its catalogue of arrangements. You must know that illness is insatiable in its demands.

Ev wakes at 6 a.m. Never have I managed to break this habit. The clock in his skinny, white body resists me. Swathed in sleep membrane he rushes in from his room across the way as if gaggles of tiny night creatures are after him. He dives in next to me in the bed, snuggles, smiles, relaxes. Such an eternal, stretching moment, long enough for you to think – will he sleep? Please – will he let me sleep? But he never does. This is a prelude. He starts to wriggle, then roll and turn, and begins to grind at my head with his rock-drill skull like a young deer with an itchy horn, at first soft and then harder, paws and toes and sharp elbows joining in, his whole body weight starting to hurt me. Closeness is not enough. To understand the mystery of my body he must gouge out a space the shape of himself inside me. As much as I love the concept of being with him in bed, I need still more to be asleep so morning always brings conflict. I am buffer and bolster between Tom and Ev. Tom's sleep is too precious to be disturbed but Tom cannot fail to be disturbed by this assault. In sleep-madness I drag Ev from the room. My mouth fills with morning bile and I hold off breakfast by force until seven. Every morning this happens.

At 9.30 a.m. sharp Mary the Physio Support worker is at the door with a folder of exercises drawn up from last week's session and a walking stick cut to Tom's height that has been produced in three days. We are impressed. She is not expected – appointments are often unscheduled – but welcome. Then at 10 a.m. Jenny and her son Alexander arrive. Alex is a forbearing seven-year-old, a good friend to Ev. He knows about guns and bombs and other things of interest. It is the school holidays and they have come round as bulk, to play with Ev and hence absorb him and us all and swell our ranks and capacity. To this end Jenny has made a handsome pie criss-crossed with filo pastry. We make an audience around the pie and marvel at it.

Now that they are here I can leave. I have chores. My tasks today are the London Library and the Mac Store. You would not believe how fast I travel. It is uncanny. I move around the city like a guided laser, so low as to be invisible. On CCTV I scarcely register. I can deviate in mid-stride, take decisions in an instant, dream in concentrated and potent segments and by 12.30 p.m. I am finished and home. Charles has brought lunch. Mary has gone so we are now six.

At 2 p.m. Dr F pops round to take some blood and make conversation. He comes often to our house and it still astonishes. We did not believe the home visit existed in this century in this city. As a GP he is an exemplar, connecting the care in the hospital to the home. Tom is dozy now, the afternoons are generally lousy for his concentration and all the others have gone out, Charles home, and Jenny and the children to the park. Ruth from the Supported Discharge Team arrives at 4 p.m. to measure up the bathroom for handrails. She has a lovely, languid manner and handles the tape measure like someone who has never seen such a thing before, waving it like a wand in the direction of things to be measured and never inclined to bend down for accuracy. She dots the tiles loosely with red crosses like kisses. Tom is asleep so he does not meet her. Alex and Jenny return with Ev, also asleep, more of a pity as it is late.

At 5 p.m. Bob turns up to try to load the voice software package I bought this morning. Tom wakes and gets involved but they can't make it work so they email a help desk in middle America with no confidence in this action. Alex and Jenny depart, leaving Ev now awake and watching a film. Just before 7 p.m. Richard arrives to deliver a painting given to us on long-term loan by an artist friend. He does not cross the threshold as he is leaving for Italy early the next day so he does not count.

Ev is now tired and grumpy and I am reading to him in bed but would prefer to be with Tom, who is still downstairs messing with the software. The doorbell rings. It is Tim on a social call, 7.30 p.m. Tim comes by nearly every day. He joins in on the software and then the reading and Ev gets a second, more animated story from him, this time with funny accents. Tim has to go. Ten minutes later Marianne comes. She is my cover for the evening. She can't resist going upstairs so Ev gets another story. He is an impossible child to refuse, a creamy and insistent lure. I go out, to do what I can't remember, and come back two hours later. Marianne leaves and then it is just the three of us again, one asleep. It is now 10 p.m. Shortly after 11 p.m. I go to sleep too, leaving Tom, whose body provides the metronome for the whole day, awake alone and ready to do some work.

2.17

How illness is transformed by technology 1.

This is the first email Tom sends to me with the help of the software package Mac Speech Dictate. It is a victorious bulletin. Tom and Tim and I are delighted with its tone of bonhomie and look forward to more.

My Dear

Team and I have made the dictate together stop it is fantastic. We will need a little bit more help to the fair and it's ROM I do mean wrong and I do not mean means to her tinnitus lofting all the time and her's basically my voice was okay for rates for the year in they sink for the basic attempt to mine to make it a service always wanted to go it but I will need a little more so goodbye for the good times he likes easy target for rubbish the

Love Tom

How illness is transformed by technology 2.

We are in the living room and Tom is trying to write an article. He works mainly in silence but when he comes to a word or phrase he cannot spell he speaks it aloud and the computer attempts to transcribe it. This is not straightforward.

In my view…

………

Basically … basically … Bay … sick … al … ee

………

Ever more so … MORE SO

………

Having … enjoying … enjoying … enjoying … oh for god's sake … enjoyed.

He is wearing headphones and speaks loudly, with emphasis. With each repetition he gets louder. I haven't got used to this and keep thinking he is speaking to me. *What's that love?*

Again … again … again … again … againnnn…

It is Beckett.

How illness is transformed by technology 3.

I am upstairs and Tom is writing downstairs. He calls me on the mobile. *But equally?* He says. *I will email you*, I say. I send an email with *But Equally* spelt out in the subject heading. He does not receive it instantly and so phones again, impatient, not wanting to wait. I send a text saying *But Equally*. The word is starting to morph as they do with repetition. Butequally. Butequally. Even I don't know what it means now though I do know how to spell it. He knows what it means though its spelling eludes him. *Thanks*, I hear faintly above the music from downstairs. Neither of us moves from our chairs.

How illness is transformed by technology 4.

The letter p has gone missing. We are in a novel by Georges Perec. Tom is trying to write the name Blue Peter. He has Blue but cannot get Peter. P. P for pasta, peach and pear. How the hell do you describe P? He never gets irate. He is infinitely patient, though our conversations over errant letters and absent words must try him as much as they do me. I nearly do not get irate either but I have many more words at my disposal and I allow my voice to rise and waste them in gabbling for solutions.

It is fantastically labour-intensive to track down a word like this. To an outsider it would be impenetrable. It would be unclear what we were doing and what exactly our problem was. *Let me try by myself*, he says, meaning, don't show me the first letter. The alphabet is written on masking tape across the top of his computer. Showing him the first letter of the word generally would solve it. *V. T. S. … No. Do you know the international alphabet call signs? P for Papa? No.* He cannot either respond to or grasp P. Then, directly, as if seized by an idea, he types into Google – *TV children's programme flag*. That he knew the double meaning of Blue Peter, both as a programme and a maritime signal, was never in doubt. That he knows how to put down these four words is secure. Blue Peter! Triumph! This is for an article on a painting by Saenredam from 1662 called *The West Front of the Sint-Mariakerk, Utrecht*. The article is completed and filed on time.

A day is only so long. It has a set amount of hours to be filled and there is Ev to think about, so the business of word finding has the power to push all else to the very edge. There is no external world: no politics, no humanitarian disasters, no murders and no scientific breakthroughs. In Chile, some miners are pulled miraculously one by one out of the earth in a tube shaped like a tampon. After that, there is only us.

2.18

Professionals are arriving in our home. They come slowly at first, in waves, but they are unstoppable. Eventually they will drown us or we will move out, whichever is the soonest. These people are the care industry and that means good and bad things. Each department on first contact brings multiple-page questionnaires and I am amazed at how sanguine Tom is in dealing with them. He is known to be easily bored and the official form is a sure trigger. He can still do sarcasm but chooses not to, and accepts the therapists, the physios and the social workers with good grace. I am beginning to understand that having people assigned to us as designated helpers is a whole area of trouble in itself. We clearly need help. Our situation might be unusual but it is not unheard of. We are a family in jeopardy and procedures are in place to deal with us, this is where the State can step in. But strangers in our home? People looking after us who do not know the heft and feel of us? I don't know what to think about this idea so I hold it at bay.

The professionals provide a new domestic audience. Will there ever be an end to the talking? Though he can make jokes about it, Tom is not yet bored with his troubles. Am I? The vagaries of his brain, nuances of speech and its lack, its many phases and quicksilver changes are always an affront. He is constantly looking for clever ways round the difficulties and the difficulties are endlessly shifting so he has to be cleverer still. It is hard sometimes to avoid the wrongheaded thought that there are two protagonists. Tom who is the master at outwitting himself, knowing as he does also when to give up and sit tight awhile, and his opponent in the grey corner – the brain – who is getting better – meaning worse – all the time: more outrageous, more merciless, more cunning. *Quicksilver* is not right in that it implies speed and to describe the processes of word finding it would be better to use local words like *mist* or *pause* or *stall* or *weave* or *grope*, none of them fast-sounding. But it is also true that there is a caprice involved, and a sleight-of-hand in some of the substitutions and in the whimsy with which things are more or less difficult or then just impossible at different times of day, struck through with occasional darts of pure accuracy. So *quicksilver* should stay.

Martin the Occupational Therapist arrives. We are impressed by him on all fronts: demeanour, body language, sense of humour and general rapport. His questions are about walking, comprehension, eating, talking, swallowing, clothes dressing, going to the toilet, fine motor skills and the exact nature of Tom's writing and how he goes about it. He wants a lot of detail. Hearing Tom's day anatomised makes me think of Richard Scarry's *Best Word Book Ever*, a great favourite with Ev and formerly of mine, particularly the double page outlining bear's dressing and breakfasting, with all the American ritual objects of the morning: pants, slippers, toothbrush, milk, maple syrup, waffles, cheerfully pictured and spelt out. If there were a question of re-learning, this book would be a useful aid. But there is no question of re-learning. This is not a rehabilitation story.

Rit. Ritard. Ritardando. The waning of Tom's ability to climb the stairs is not sequential but like a single protracted event unfolding over time. The stairs to the bedrooms on the top floor are irregular and steep. I gauge by ear the long and longer pauses between footfalls. The structure of the house, its joists and the creak of the wooden treads record and amplify the effort. How many months have I been listening in this way? I hear it most clearly when Tom comes up after me as I lie in bed and I know that if Ev is awake, he hears it too. My heart thumps. It is fat. My head fills with blood. I am an animal that knows its own end and is poised, ready to jump. *Will he make it?* The heart pushes against the chest wall and at the turn of the stair at the top, the last step the hardest, relaxes again. He always makes it. He does not fall. Only when of his own volition he decides to stop trying, only when that day comes, do we make a bed for him on the floor below. If I can interpret the slowness of this passage on the stairs then Ev can do it too. I never underestimate Ev's intelligence. If I do, I am always proved wrong.

Martin is part of the external team bringing handrails, bath seats and bed raisers into our lives. He works closely with Tom to find ways of putting the wayward physical strength of his body to best use. On our bed Martin models for Tom the standard technique for getting out of bed without undue strain. Tom tries this but cannot do it at all and thinks it is very funny. He then shows Martin his own improvised method for getting up. The starting posture is lying down on his back with legs bent, hands clasped tightly together as if on a rock-face, hanging on to an imaginary rope for dear life and then a great rocking haul see-sawing along the spine that sends him by will and momentum up into a sitting position. I have seen this many mornings past. It is so counter-intuitive that Martin has not seen anything like it and he tries it himself but cannot do it for laughing. Then I try. They are both laughing. In a sun-shower of dust motes we repeat our absurd rehearsal. *Action 1. Getting out of bed.*

That our house is not a bungalow but a maisonette on three floors with a total of three staircases containing thirty-eight steps from top landing to pavement outside is what you might call a bad hand. When we bought it we had the fancy that the top floor with the study and half the books was for Tom. The middle one with the kitchen, living room and three sofas was mine. The draughty hall below containing the rest of the books was where Ev would live quietly with his toys. Three people in harmony: one on each floor. In reality Ev has the top, middle and the bottom and we live around his rim.

Tom is speaking well today even though it is 2 p.m., generally his worst time. He is enjoying Martin's company and his line of questions and appreciates the fact that they travel readily further than the subject. Martin does the physical too. I have watched this many times. *Push against my hand, hard as you can. Pull my arms towards you. Can you touch your nose and then my finger? Good. Good. Touch each finger in sequence with your thumb. Can you screw up your eyes tight? Good. Great.* One day, I think. One day you may not be able to touch the finger with your finger and it will hover blankly in the air or you will miss your own nose on the return. I may witness this but I hope I do not.

In homemade parallel with Martin and the actions of Social Services we put our faith in the ingenuity of friends for the intimate workings of our life. Our home is being adapted headlong without pause for assessment or breath. We have rails and grips dotted around the house courtesy of the Social, but Health and Safety is their charter and Tom is finding the step and turn from the landing into the bedroom resistant. It is bitter. He has not the pull in his arms to draw up his body nor the traction in his thigh to make the stair. We need a handle on the bedroom door and the door must be fixed back to take his weight. This is too complex for the State. We move at speeds faster than it can think. So John brings his toolbox over to research this and other domestic snags – the top of the stairs, the three steps in the hall, the height of the bed. Tom and John investigate each point of flash and fail and at each one John installs a handle or a block fixed rock-solid as an abseil anchor by a seasoned mountaineer. All of these hurdles need addressing as soon as they arise. *Action 2. Entering the bedroom.* It is imperative, simply the practice of living. Otherwise we will fall. We do not say, John and I, though we know, that these solutions are transient as the days of the week. The fixing is in opposition to the ephemerality of the problem. The problem will worsen and soon. The solution is its own redundancy. The solidity of the fixing is the entire rebuke to this fact.

And so the days go; single, horizontal days, each a sheet of picture glass. It is possible to work for a fortnight on a solution that is used once. Or for a week on a clever piece of ingenuity that becomes unviable three days before it is implemented. We live in hyper-inflation. Our efforts double one day, and again the next. As all work is folly, we just work harder. On the phone I price up stair lifts. Tom is keen. A lift would help him a great deal. But it would help him now, today, on *this* climb of the stair. I can hazard nothing about what will help him in three months by the time it is installed.

Ever so lightly we are balanced and the balance holds as long as we look neither forward nor back. The fulcrum is the world. And right into these precarious days, upheld by an ad-hoc army of logistical support, comes the implementation of the Social Services care package. To an observer our situation must look perilous. Now it tips into catastrophe. I see it coming but I sleepwalk towards this intervention. The argument as given to me is circular, meaningless, a tautology. *Something must be done*/I have no other solution/*You need help*/This is not a solution/*Something must be done* ...

Tom is assigned carers. They come for half an hour, three times a day, three days a week and a key safe is added to our porch so that strangers can let themselves in. I work hard to keep Ev out of it. I know it won't be pretty. Even on paper the plan looks unworkable and I book them in for days when Ev is at nursery. The carers are not uniformly bad but they are not uniformly anything and they multiply exponentially the things I have to fear. In thirty-minute clocked slots we must get to know them and they us. If all the clients were fish, we might be fed and have our tanks cleaned out in this time. There is no investment within the schedule in learning Tom's needs. The system allows no time. On the care schedule we are compressed by paper jargon to the point of idiocy. The list is an arbitrary work of directives. *Point 13. Settle the client in front of the television.* It is fiction.

Some of the carers I warm to as much as I can, Claire, Barbara, Yusuf, but I never know when they will come again. Insecurity fuels the system. I cannot attest to their characters or trust when they will arrive, or if they will arrive at all. The only uniformity is in the paucity of their training and remit. The stated aim of the care package is to take the pressure off me and allow me the freedom to leave the house. Instead I must entrench. I am the last line of defence.

After the second week I am preparing to cancel. I cannot bear it. This is the thing that will destroy us. Through these two years, our autonomy has been a closely loved and guarded miracle. We have not been damaged. We are impregnable still. Now, the heart of who we are is under attack. Cancer has not managed to do this. This is going to be done by people. One of the carers talks to Tom loudly as if he is senile. One wakes him, ignoring the poster-sized note I leave on the door asking her please not to. One does not know his name. One bangs the door hard downstairs on her way out. The lock is capricious. She does not look behind her and leaves the door standing open to the street.

I am upstairs, but a while later I come down to get something. The hall is splashy with light and a fine breeze refreshes my face. Autumn soaks the street and shadows of leaves invade the mat. All is abundant. To every problem we think of a way forward but the unforeseen is increasing steadily in its mass. Now I see it in plain sight. If I had not been here anyone could have come in. Tom would have been alone. We are breached. Something has entered. I am weightless and without hunger. All our vulnerability swoops into the hall, filling it, squeezing me out. The air flickers, alive with its spirit presence. Sunlight licks the walls and laps over the floor towards my bare feet. At our door is the world's brim. We are wide open. There is nothing between us and nothing.

The next morning, when I wake, I see lights at the far corner of my eyes. White, warning flashes I cannot control are exploding on the edges of my vision.

2.19

We go to the community garden but without Tom. A little pattern is emerging. It is clear how it goes. People come to see him, spend time with him and then at some point signal that they want to scurry off with me for a private talk about his condition. He cannot, as they say, give them much change for their money at the moment. He is just too tired. I had better get used to this, though it is new and it feels like a fresh betrayal. I am becoming Tom's mouth. Without being Tom's brain I am clearly a fraud, and people who try to come to him through me are bound to be disappointed.

The community garden was once the nursery for the old house that sits at the high point of the park. It is still partially surrounded by the original brick wall, some 20m high, and the bones of all that was there, the cold frames, greenhouses, paths and orchard, have been picked over and reconstituted by the volunteers who have maintained it for the last two decades in a testament to altruism and anarchy, long-term common interests, mistakes left to lie and a multitude of digging hands. It is accurately named and a crowded knowledge of horticulture is visible all around, coupled with an unplanned waywardness, the plants a bohemian set, all thick with each other.

On the outside the park grass slopes away stubby as clipped straw, but the municipal parch stops neatly at the gate and the earth within the garden is madly verdant, fuelled by three small hills of high-grade mulch near the entrance in order of increasing potency and slippage. This afternoon the sky is slate, heavy with rain. Its tone pre-sets all the colours within the walls to full saturation. Giant ricin sprouts wine-red and black behind the beans. Every angle is askance, every path wobbles and edges are demarcated with tile, pot, brick, pebble, shell, wood, whatever, with no pattern ever repeated, no line continuous with another. Signs are written in wetted marker pen. CRAFTS it says, upside down. Cucumber tendrils spiral freehand through the roof space of the greenhouse. Yellow courgette flowers and gourds of a day-glo hue thrive on wet bales of hay sunk into pits and the growing of peppers, maize and chillies of many varieties and strengths is a local pride. I wonder that I have not spent more time here. It is spectacular. The orchard has old pear, medlar, quince, apple and other fruits we cannot name though my friends have more knowledge than I. In a magic realist enclave, a travelling camp of runner beans twists up to bind the tree canopy above to the ground below, their lines fretted by strings of silver can lids. The late, humid air is spiked with herbs brushed and mashed by the day's visitors. We sit on planks by the pond in the wild seed section, planted tight like everything else and fully wild to a dimension of 2 square metres. All is arranged like crazy paving; the yellow, the red, the bark, the tile, the brick, the black, the pot, the plank, and I look at it in a kind of blankness, barely present in body but really I am taking in all of it in detail as if to memorise it for another.

There is seeing and there is telling and what is one without the other? In a marriage of near ten years and a friendship of longer, all visual experience is for two. To see something is to store it up even as it is happening, as potential news, not even news, sub-news, to be retold, embellished, filtered or censored and described to another. The other. This is not conscious but directly continuous with experience so it is light work; banal, beautiful, boring, it makes no matter. We both do it. It is the story of what we see and do when we are apart from each other gifted back in fragments. I assume others do it too.

Not immediately but maybe much later, something will emerge and be presented with no great authority, like the gift of a nut, or a crisp, a small twist of paper, a bit of wool, perfect for the time and recipient. These low gifts are indiscriminate, you can never have too many of them. *He will like this.* They don't hold the status of gossip or anything particularly interesting but are just a bit of the world in the right ear.

Choose your moment. *I saw this in the community garden.* The world experienced is the world described. This retelling in turn is such an intimate pleasure and so deep in the muscle of seeing and following on from that, of being. Soon, sometime soon I will have no one to tell this to. What will experience be then?

2.20

I notice that we haven't talked for a while. How long? An hour? It may be normal. Sometimes you just don't.

There are general issues of talking and beyond that there is the Talking Issue, meaning talking about what is going on, articulating the disaster that coagulates around us. Tom promised a while back to begin a conversation with Ev and he has not done this. I try to give him a chance. It is not my place to pre-empt with explanations but perhaps he cannot and will not ever, so I must. He is stumbling over the pronunciation of bedtime stories. *Get into your teeth*, he says to Ev, meaning *Get into your bed.* I feel that Ev needs to start being given a version of our narrative that he can make sense of himself: a nuanced, acclimatising story with a ready line to follow. How that story goes and what it sounds like I am not sure but it won't be like the ones in his books. There will be no happy end, no moral neatness, no rhyme. Pictures aplenty though. We make images all the time. I take the photographs. Ev lying on Tom's fat stomach, Ev spooning in cereal while Tom drinks a slow tea. Us three idling down the road as usual. I feel that two adults must be intelligent enough and brave enough to come up with something here, some version of a story to help Ev negotiate it. So far I am wrong.

I realise that I am still imagining a canny way by which we will manage when Tom can no longer communicate. That some sub-route will open up to bypass all language, spoken and written, and allow us still to converse. How will this go? Does a raised eyebrow conform to a conversation? What will be the modes available? Touch, sight, laughter, will there be any of that? We expect a great deal of each other. The tools we have are steadily depreciating. We must use these poor, truncated tools or create new ones from scratch.

Silences hold more pressure. It is simply more difficult to form and find words. We have had a weekend of heavy socialising and I watch Tom all eager, talking in a mix of fluid, lucid, stalled and jumbled speech. When he is with me he needs to recuperate from the effort and this can mean he is quiet and I don't get spoken to. I understand the toll of each conversation but I am jealous. The oddest word-slips emerge. Logs becomes otters. *Ev went round the park treading on the otters*. I notice that I too muddle words and things come out wrong. This is an empathetic response, automatic, like my not so appealing habit of faintly echoing the accent of the person I am speaking to.

Since the second operation and considerably over the last days he has become more introspective. There are wider silences. We are slower together. When he is with me I feel his absence. I say this but cannot calibrate it. I don't have the statistics. Is this person quieter than they were yesterday? Is he starting conversations or is it always me who begins? Is he spending more time by himself? How long is it since he spoke? Is there anything to say?

This is impossible. I am tuning myself to detect quietness, to monitor changes in sub-patterns and catch the point when silence starts. I am alive to change yet I am nowhere near a sensitive enough instrument to record it. I have empirical evidence but cannot interpret the data. How to separate companionable silence from withdrawal? What if it is just not necessary to add anything more? He and his brain are one. That means that he and the cancer in his brain are one, having lived together for nearly two years. They know each other well. My watchfulness is as much about me as about him. I am angry. How dare he vanish from my side. In order to support him I must have something in return and companionship is the whole of my demand. I see the idiocy of it. But this new silence feels cruel and personal. It is a further blow. It takes me a couple of days, a little time, just a little, to allow the thought that introspection, aloneness, set-apartness, might be in order after brain surgery. To be quiet in the privacy of one's own head, surely this is a good thing.

I have a text draft permanently on my phone. *All ok? x*, it says. I use it hourly when apart from him. The reply comes, *x*, or *Yes*. All the time around the house although I try to limit my vigilance, whenever I see him sitting or gazing out the window I catch myself asking, *Are you all right, sweet?* I do this until I realise there is something important I have forgotten. This is what he most liked to do anyway. Thinking. Repose. Regeneration. He wrote an article on it once after Pascal. It was called *In praise of sitting quietly in my room. I am thinking.* He says, *I am just thinking.* I must let him be. I must just let the man be.

Yet wordlessness can be exquisite. There are times when Tom can speak when we have nothing more to say. The car is a natural arena for this. It is a luxury to sit next to each other in silence. Returning at night from somewhere, I park outside our house and we sit awhile with the headlights on. It is better if it is raining. The bark of the birch tree to the right glows luminous. When I turn the lights off, the after-image of the tree remains as an elegant smear of oily white like a line of paint. We sit and we are silent. Rain patterns the road and dins on the car roof. This sight is so near, so familiar that the road smudging into darkness takes our thoughts with it. We live in real time. Here we are in our car. This is the street outside our house. This is where we live.

2.21

I would tell you about the camaraderie of the chemo day room but today we have the wrong attitude, so it is not working and for the first time the reverse is happening. We are getting on people's nerves. A lady with a leathery tan and her silent husband opposite disapprove of us. They have come prepared and are settled in already like promenaders at the Royal Albert Hall, habitués with flasks and newspapers, taking positions well in advance and assured in their intimate knowledge of the way things go. We are clearly making far too much fuss and showing our discontent. Perhaps that's not done. Mostly we take the drugs at home as pills. But it's not even that we are new to this, we have been here before; sitting, waiting, saline flushing, but something is askew. The micro-workings of the chemotherapy machine, the innards of its outlandish system, have got clagged up and mired in psychological sand. Tom is tired and therefore less coherent. It is the worst time of day for him to be out and it's dawning on us that we have been called here in optimism well in advance of anything happening. Only after an hour and a half of waiting do the cytotoxics arrive on a trolley in thrice-checked, light-resistant sealed packets. The chemo room is several staff members short so the delay looks set to expand in all directions.

Smiley nurse on secondment comes up. *My, you look tired*, she says brightly to me. *I have been here for an hour and half with nothing happening. I need to get home in time to collect my child from nursery and today is my birthday.* Tom doesn't believe in not complaining and I have learnt some useful lessons over the years in the straight art. I have got much better at it. Smiley nurse is now repeating at us, *Have you got a line? Have you got a line? A line?* She is pointing at Tom. We are puzzled and frayed like foreigners at customs. Tom asks for the music to go down so that he can make sense of her. *Sweet dreams are made of this. Who am I to disagree ...* Tan lady tuts and rustles her crossword. After a minute says in a measured tone to the room, *It's the worst thing, to not be able to quite hear the radio.* I look at her. *Do turn it up now if you want to. He just couldn't hear. It doesn't matter*. She does not reply, her eyes snap down to her paper, 3 down, *bovine*, and won't meet mine. They never do meet mine. It is all a bit like being on a long bus ride but with drugs. There are the usual boredoms and embarrassments, minor aggro. The passengers are here but not here, on their way somewhere else, in the world or out of it.

The room is more or less empty and all during our non-encounter with tan lady the man in the corner chair is staring at me. I meet his eye once and decide not to do so again. He is looking with bright interest, as an entomologist looks at a beetle. When not looking at us he seems to be asleep or resting, his head tilted back discreetly, but when alert, his blue-grey eyes are fixed on us. He is in his late sixties, aggressively neat with his shirt a bright ironed white and cuffs turned up over his arm, with the line – now I know what this is – perforating his wrist as it lies lightly across a pillow on his knee. He may be an habitué but he is a quiet one, without books or papers. Our minor commotions seem to be his only interest. His hair is a shade yellower than his shirt but not by much. His face is chalk white.

To distract us, I sit with my mouth close to Tom's ear and read poems in a low voice that slips below the beeping of the drips and the teeny, tinny, too-quiet radio: a rubbish one by Hardy, Auden's *The Fall of Rome*, a Larkin something or other. It really is my birthday. I don't care that much but grim just the same.

In 1865 the photographer Edward Fox took two pictures. Together as a document they make an elegant pair of brackets. One is *Chestnut (Spanish) in Winter, Buxted Park, Sussex.* The other, *Chestnut (Spanish) in Summer, Buxted Park, Sussex,* is taken from exactly the same point. Between them, the photograph I want to see does not exist. It would show the point of turn.

Is it possible as a form of record to know how long a tree takes to lose its leaves? It may start in late summer, say, August. It would depend on the type. What would be the average for a municipal elm in the park at Kennington soaked at the base in dog and human wee, its roots infiltrating drains and each leaf drawing fumes deep into the vessels and knots of the wood? And would it be slower then for an old oak at Selborne, Hampshire, high on the weald, exposed to smashes of wind and violent shifts of air? How long would each take to drop and become the outline of its own skeleton? Can this be charted?

Leaves are the talkers and the articulators of shape, the shifting thrill and shrill of the tree, the noise. How long do you think? I want to know. I understand there are many parameters – vagaries of aspect, wind, weather, disease, drought or seasonal shift. But when might you notice the first one falling? Who is to record it? Who will catch it as it sidles down, not just a rogue leaf but a marker, the signal of the real turn. Autumn, Fall, is now. So it is with us, from August this year and ongoing, Fall is now.

Back at home we have a long talk. This is our favourite activity. I don't even think about how incredible it is that we can do it still. The place to do it is on the sofa, now jacked up on blocks so that Tom can get up and down more easily and blockaded beneath with a barrier of the fattest art books; Uffizi and Pitti complete, Hermitage, Vatican, Louvre, National Gallery, Musée d'Orsay entire. The books make an institutional barricade. Each is about 12 cm thick and they stop Ev disappearing under the sofa in curls of dust and broadband cable. Tom is laughing. *You are so good – how you undercept me*. He is brilliant at this; his hybrid of understand and intercept is exactly right. I can pick up his meaning prior to understanding, near pre-articulation. I can sometimes get in there so fast I am his mouth and message. This is why I will not leave him alone now, in case I miss something, a phrase that it might grieve me not to hear.

Our friends don't want to leave him alone either. The house is full of people: sitters, supporters, cooks, companions and watchers just in case. He is the motor for all this and drives it with urgency: more, more. The last time we came out of hospital I wanted us to have a couple of days' rest to acclimatise to home and to Ev, but no. The next morning at ten we were at the table working on the article he was writing, the one about language and illness, picking at his notes, guessing, finding, repeating, hammering at every word until we got there.

Now. I think I need to say it now, he says. I have paper and a pen. I am ready. *I want four things*. He has done his homework and in his notebook he has written down these words not really as words but as rubbings of them, bundles of letters, tracks and caches of lines done so lightly in pencil. He shows me. He cannot say them but I can decipher them. They are, *Speech? Quiet but still something? Noises? Nothing*? He is precise. Here are four stages in order, as accurate as he can make them. Recorded from within.

Halfway through the work he breaks off. *What is this lump*? A small hill is rising on the side of his head at the site of the scar. I touch it with my finger. A thing. I had noticed it first a few days previous hidden under his hair but definitely it seems bigger. It is growing. We are puzzled. We think of the skull like a motorbike helmet that can shatter but not expand. We mark it down to tell Dr B at the next clinic. *What is this*? Her fingers go to it quickly, gently parting the hair. Her eyes narrow.

2.22

Lasagne, chicken with couscous, lemon cheesecake, a pork and bacon pie, lentil soup, a three-tier blueberry cake, ready-made meals for kids, pasta sauce, half a chicken, beetroot and apple salad, rhubarb fool, sausage rolls, ham, macaroni cheese, clafoutis, fish pie, bread pudding, figs, shepherd's pie, lamb casserole, a whole chicken, roast chicory, spinach and chickpea tart, bolognaise sauce, rice salad, chestnut and celeriac soup, hummus, spicy chicken wings, croissants, beef stew, bread, vitello tonnato, caramelised onion tart, duck, peaches, a great deal of cheese, a basket of little cakes anointed.

Friends have been bringing food to our door over the last two years. Often they stay to eat with us but not always. Praise for the foods and praise for the bringers of foods.

2.23

Plasticity. This is the environment we live in. It is volatile and dangerous. Our family is a working model of the plasticity of the brain. Tom's consciousness is doing a barely-checked work of unpicking itself. Dishevelment is the order of the day; of edges, surfaces, nuances, formulations, habits. Yesterday his voice went funny, not his language but his speaking voice, and he spoke like a person thick-tongued and cartoon stupid. Yet this does not hold true this morning and it may not be true tomorrow. *I don't like how my voice sounds*, he grumbles, *it's ugly*. We could be a controlled experiment on flux and micro-change, on plasticity in action. Scientists could come and live with us over forty-eight hours, connect us to a three-way monitor. We have a spare room. They could set up their equipment there. I shall apply for a Wellcome Grant. I got money before, only a couple of years ago – so short? – in another life, for a film they commissioned. I filmed objects from their collection and laid them out on a black ground. I filmed them like you could feel them, pick them up and stroke them and then in intervals of black, each like a long shutter, one would slip its moorings and change places with another. It was about the paying of close attention, about touch and the lovely redundancy of filming the inanimate: duration stripped of agency. Nothing much happened. With us, much too much is happening. Our lives are live streamed and no one is in charge.

Come ladies and gentlemen scientists, come record the words running into each other and garbling, regard the thoughtfulness of Ev as he watches and listens even when appearing not to do so, chart the surges, the rallies and the minor collapses, photograph the way I hold my body in extreme watchfulness and note how I never actually rest. Test the blood sugar of the group at various times of day, map my eye movements as they run over any given hour, monitor the ways in which our hearts beat separate and together, count the number of times I shout *You all right, love*? and note from which rooms I tend to shout it and how high my voice is pitched. Come and chart us for the record. Tom has been asleep for two days solid and the last two nights I have taken to sleeping with Ev. It is a single bed. This feels temporary but extraordinarily relaxing. This is what can happen in a domestic family when the normal formulation of cells is interrupted.

We are in a highly polarised situation. Tom is being here linguistically unformed yet he is moving like an adventurer into ever rarer territory and working hard at it while Ev pursues its straight opposite, bashing away merrily like a junior workman with a Fisher-Price tool-box. He is fearless and jovial, learning to craft language even as he is not sure what it means. Both are engaged in a work of beyond-the-brink resourcefulness, an improvisatory balancing act, an enforced making up as they go along. Tom is an inventor, an innovator, a pioneer, as is Ev. Both of them are on the front line of personhood, more so now than ever.

Ev's brain is of course as impressionable as dough, as clever as – there is nothing cleverer than a child on accelerated learning. Today was his first day at big nursery. *Blue-goo on your head. Blue-goo poo on you*, said Ev when he came home. He may not say this again. Blue-goo with glitter in it was a substance from little nursery and he has moved on and left Blue-goo behind. Information goes in to be parked against other bits of information, shelved and saved for later, unregarded, waiting to be made sense of or used.

I watch him in the playground forging neural pathways as he shoots tinted water along the bamboo gutter. He notes that it will go downhill and not up and constructs ever more complex runnels and routes, wetting his shorts and shoes and cuffs – how children hate wet cuffs.

I hear him mobilising the meanings of words as he says *Have you ever seen a combine harvesting the rain?* He understands from somewhere that rain might be likened to stalks of wheat, that combine-harvester has a verb in it that may be adapted, that the impossible might be addressed directly through speech, and that chasms and categories of ideas can be skipped over and bounced on. In words! Only words. This is pure play, pleasure and pastime, done just for the hellery. His visual intelligence keeps pace with his linguistic advances. He presents me with two empty Evian bottles side by side on the table, a litre one and a half litre one. *This one is Dad and this is me.*

The brain is said to never cease its work of adjustment in the normal run of a life. In our family experiment I would ask the ladies and gentlemen scientists to take a look at mine. It feels as if it has changed state and been thrice cooked. It is not remotely plastic or adaptable or clever, nothing like dough or some zippy modern moulding medium, but is more materially akin to an obscure man-made and obsolescent substance like Bakelite between the wars; brittle, chipped, hard, yellowing, nearing the end of its life.

2.24

My love is cryptic. He speaks in mysteries. He speaks a language that is singular. Communication with Tom is nothing like speaking any other language. It is at the same time known by heart and deeply foreign.

Late in the day (*Why did they leave it so late?* you cry) we are trying to elide language altogether and invent a communication that bypasses all known words. We do not have a lot of time. We do not sign and are not so stupid as to learn. The brain orchestrates the hands. You cannot teach the fingers autonomy like a little manual dance troupe. No, the language we are looking for must circumnavigate the brain. (You laugh.) How clever it is. How hard we try to outwit it. How it foils us. In an open folly Tom makes a wild attempt on language one morning in the kitchen. His plan is to use colour, and to demonstrate he takes the set of melamine side-plates. This one (red) means this, this one (olive) means this, this one (grey) means this, this one (saffron) means this. We look at each other unconvinced. The set of all known things you might want to say maps nowhere on to a suite of nine coloured discs.

After discussion we arrive at a word list, though we both know this may not help and indeed is not likely to help, but we assemble a list of topics by way of a start point. The plan is to head off subjects, cut down on the guessing of desires and things and narrow the verbal field. Our list is made of the current main themes arising. I print it out in *Gill Sans* and stick it on the wall, where it will stay for months. When words go I will voice each item and pray that the matter in hand pertains to one of them. If it does not then we are dumped back in the linguistic vastness beyond the list. The list seems narrow and though you might say as an observer that our field of operation is narrowing all the time, it doesn't feel like that at all to us. We are in a formless, live state that changes daily, spreading and pooling like a poured liquid of strange viscosity left unchecked; at once broader and more saturated than we ever were before.

MEDICAL CARE
WRITING AND WORK
MY COMPUTER
FUN THINGS TO DO
MY BODY
AFTER MY DEATH
MARION
EV
FOOD
CLOTHES
FRIENDS
MUSIC
PICTURES
THE OUTDOORS
READING
POETRY

The immediate problem is that I am becoming the whole of the context. The swiftest way to cut to the chase with Tom – and of course, that's what many want to do, privileging arrival/comprehension over the journey/experience – is to talk to me. This is by no means true of all and we have a solid core of those who stay and spend the time it takes – for really if you are going to join with us, this is the life and it will use all the time you give it. These last weeks since when I can't remember we have been working at words around the clock. We all do it, solo and in small groups at a time. Collectively we are his amanuenses and close workers on text. Tom has projects he wants to see made public. He is the editor. His back catalogue is vast and protean. Our job is to organise his thoughts and writings under dictation. We rewrite under instruction, calibrate what's important, flesh out structures and crucially note where all the stuff is on the computer. Only when I sleep does this stop and when I wake up it starts again. It is exhilarating, satisfying, frustrating and it is *my* work. After one particularly arduous session, hammering over and over at points I suspect we will go over again tomorrow, Tom looks at me. It has been a good session. He is delighted, amused, he says. *Ultimately, you will know everything.*

As someone who writes for newspapers, Tom's language will survive beyond the ephemeral. One book project is in the making. We have a publisher and are moving towards a date. Others are forming and their nebulous state now that they have been articulated is tantalising. His words have always read deceptively easy on the page, echoing his conversational, deep speaking voice. Here they are being made ready. Here are the things that will come into being. They represent a future.

At the end of this month his piece will appear in the *Observer*: summoning his situation in 5,000 clear and precise words, not posthumously as a ghost but as a man observing himself living under great duress. It is a work on language and much else besides, described from the epicentre of a storm. His wayward lexicon is of primary concern and he is ever occupied with the gradations and nuances of his writing. It has to be right. This is what concerns him in composing the article. He gets me to arrange the phrases. He always was a perfectionist: alert to touch and beat and tone and still is the same but the tools are infinitely slippery and weightless, like beads of mercury. This is the article we finish in these violent days on the cusp of everything collapsing and it is a group finish. We are elated as drunks. For weeks his words have been read aloud in the house like an epic poem. I expect Ev to know them by heart and say them back to me in years to come.

He would always speak his writing out. Late at night I used to hear it, a man declaiming loudly under his breath so as not to disturb us: checking the words, their good action, testing them to see if they go well to the reader. The mind is an organ of hearing. The word is the sound of the word. Words have been shepherded out, spoken and found to be good. They are exactly the ones he wants to use and as his judgement was always so precise there is no reason to doubt it now. He is printed, he is written down. That's this week's success. What will happen next week? And that is public but what of our private language? How can a language endure if it has only one to speak it and another to give it context? We are a people of two and ours is a dying tongue. Our plight may be picked up and our conversation studied by a researcher in an East Coast University, the results analysed, digitised, archived.

Waiting in clinic Tom asks me to make a list of the names of all his friends and what they are. This is puzzling. I try to ascertain if I am to write a minute pen portrait of each and almost make a start as it could be fun, an opportunity for simple wickedness, but no. Finally we arrive at what he wants and as so often it is much simpler than I might have imagined, being a list of their name and surname. It starts with us, Tom, Ev and me without our afternames, and then the rest follow in a raggedy line. He cannot do names now, sometimes not the first one or the second or both and even though he knows their faces and is sure about their dearness to him, the lack of title is discomfiting and puts him on more of a back foot than he is already. He is unhappy that his grasp of my name too is fluctuating. I say I don't care what name he calls me by – and there are a few – because I am always certain that it is me he knows. Tom's confusion is linguistic. It is neither emotional nor intellectual.

Next, I am asked to write down a list of opposites. *Dark – Light. Big – Small. Yes – No. High – Low. Full – Empty*. We have done this before and I know he tried it himself in a notebook some weeks previously. As I write these and say them aloud he is fascinated and says, *Ah yes, that's an interesting one*. But today, unusually, his reading is coming down each time to one pairing, the root pair it seems, and every pair he reads he voices only as BIG – SMALL. *Big – Small*, said each time with different emphasis and stress and enormous gusto as if each was a different word entirely. It is as if the meaning and import of all the other words – *fast–slow*, *wide–narrow*, *light–heavy* – is retained in the style and manner of the articulation of the root pair while only *it* can be actually spoken. Names – friends – opposites. His interest in all this is genuine and his excitement is infectious. As I write I lean against him like a sandbag. Skipping over the content it is fun and we pass the time well and companionably. I can feel humour sidling up in the words and in the inflection of his voice: the up pair, the down pair, the fat pair, the lean pair, the full pair, the empty.

So this is how it is. As I said: no optimism, no content, no publication, no orchestra, no ladder but now fleshed out. Many of his words are gone, words which mean things, words which mean people, words for food, for clothes, for trees, for jobs, for countries, pronouns, adverbs, verbs, nouns. *The subject, sweetheart*, I am always saying, *what's the subject*?

A conversation earlier went like this.

What's the subject? Are you talking about your work?

A little bit more.

Your writing?

Little bit more.

Your whole life?

Little bit less.

We never get to the bottom of that one. What is left is the connective tissue of conversation. *Something like that. On the one hand on the other hand. All this over there*, said with a swoop of the hand, means the world outdoors. Intelligence powers speech. Even when we can't talk, it is all we do. Sometimes I pray for silence. We loop and loop in wide, hilarious conversations that either get there in the end or are terminally derailed and come to rest on high ground. These conversations depend on a focused companion mind ready to go outside all the beaten tracks and desire lines. If I have the patience, and mainly I do unless tiredness knocks me out of the ring, I can fuel this stuff for hours. Some friends are brilliant at it. Others don't grasp what's going on and what is required of them. They can't do it at all.

With our friends at their house we sit for an evening and ramble till its end. Tonight the topics include Adam Philips – whose book Tom reviewed not so long ago, aspects of high-level curatorial appointments, how to curtail a child's play from taking over the house, an acquaintance we have in common, the remodelling of a gallery (our friend is an architect), Tom's language – even he is a bit bored by talking about this – and food. As ever he gets stuck into the heart of it. All conversing goes via him. He never sits out. So a conversation then, but every named thing in it: architect, gallery, Lego, philosopher, sex, book, salami, has to be reached on a discursive journey through fantastical strings of yes/no questions, huge circuits of expanded guesswork in long baggy primary trails which drag their own secondary subjects into the open. While we talk, we drink, and I see that on the side he is doing tiny scruffy, spidery drawings with great care, rubbed out and runic and set out in diagrammatic relationships to each other: a tree, a knot, a clock face, a computer, a typewriter, pictograms drawn in pencil waiting to have words attached to them. These are unlike anything he has done before and I can see by his concentration that it is an attempt at a new mode. Pressed against his shoulder I know he is relaxed and enjoying himself immensely in exactly the way he would have enjoyed such an open-ended gossipy evening years ago.

I have been gifted but the gift is perhaps the same as a lack. It is to feel neither horror nor pity. Sadness yes, and a sort of intractable physical weight at the impossible hand with Ev aged three and Tom near fifty-three. But this is us. This is how we are and that fact makes everything much easier. How may I feel pity for us? There exists no objective view. Seen from where I am, we are great. We always have been. Ev's push-along zebra finally enters the conversation without

Tom being able to say any of these words: zebra, animal, child, toy, wheel, wood.

2.25

In the consulting room of the diabetes nurse Tom looks very sick. The lighting is aggressive and I see him clearly for the first time in days. Though bright, our house is nowhere so evenly lit as this. The morning sun at full shout filters through large windows filmed with dust and historic rain. We are both wearing the clothes we got up in not very long ago and Tom looks eroded and shabby around the edges. He is a big, dark garden rose blown out at the end of season, a hybrid, purple and black. His eyes are dulled. His hair is damp with sweat.

His silhouette was always dynamic, strangely elastic and crisp for a large man, and kept its energy well. Now he seems loose, his flesh not kempt but wayward, no longer trimmed in tight by the body's pull. Forces other than gravity are at work. Gravity drags down while cancer pushes out from the centre. It is a centrifugal disease that screws up everything: hair, eyes, legs, teeth, nails, bones, feet. Struwwelpeter: a malign force. I suspect that I look quite bad in this light too.

Diabetes has developed as a result of long-term steroid use. It is just one of those extra, unexpected things, like epilepsy and oedema and fatigue, which if you were at all medical you would know about readily but if not you find out incompetently and by degrees. We are under some pressure to take it seriously and we sort of do but not very, not with the hand we hold. Diabetes just gives us a deal more hassle.

In clinic, under these conditions – first thing in the morning, we are dead on our feet – Tom's regard for diabetes as a topic is low, and bored by the fussing of the nurse he blanks out and drifts. His stare hovering to my left is static. I see that stare more and more these days and keep having to call him back to me. *I'm over here*. Because before we were proximate even when apart, I cannot just let this go. Sometimes I wave as if from a shore. I understand this stare to mean either that he cannot quite follow us or that we are talking too fast. But a more optimistic take – maybe quite accurate – would be that his mind is still his own. He is taking up the precious seconds he needs to use it. He knows I can do the diabetes stuff, so he doesn't have to.

I observe him. Is he going to fall over? I wonder. He hasn't yet, but might at any point. Is he asleep? Will he be able to get out of that chair again? Getting out of a chair is a complex muscular action that his legs and forearms strain to do. He is a dying man. That is what he looks like. How long has his skin been this pale yellowish-grey? It's as pale as joiner's putty or porcelain unfired.

Then I realise that the others in the room, Dr F and the diabetes nurse, are thinking the same thing as me. I notice how Dr F hovers slightly behind him on the balls of his feet with his palms splayed open, alert to any small, unreliable shifts in the upper body that might signify the beginning of a topple with gravity pulling him unresisting down from the chair like a statue from a plinth. I would sympathise with a fall. You could fall through plain boredom. The will to lie on the floor, to be carted off somewhere else and dealt with, has a strong attraction. I feel it too.

In clinic our conversation has moved subtly over the hour from talking to Tom as a patient, to talking about him. We talk over him and he signals that he allows this. My view shifts the longer we are here. I have crossed over. I see him almost from the outside. I am a participant and he is not. Later, I have a conversation with the oncologist, Dr B. *He is likely to become more withdrawn*, she says … *to take less and less part in things. This can seem to those close to a patient like the most disturbing thing. This is the brain protecting itself.* This is not at all how it goes.

Certain words are creeping into my vocabulary. Single words and phrases like flag-bearers for my new narrative. They come slow, like a procession of mourners. *Carer* is one I resist. *Palliative* another. *Single parent* – I never voice it but it is the case. *Terminal*. I never, ever, say this though I know its ambit. *Brain damage*. No – neither. These are not new concepts, but I have hesitated a long while now and they have not been assigned a place. Doing is one thing. Doing is easy frankly, certainly easier than the other thing, which is to give a thought a name.

To word a thought: this is a subtle and evasive thing for Tom. For me, with certain words it is a conscious aggression against myself. Retrospective naming, speaking a thing aloud once you have long got used to it and worn it in, that's the softer way. I forgive myself such elisions because it works. I can be several paces ahead, my mind on something else entirely when suddenly struck; I turn and see the thing clear behind me and call out. *There!* I act surprised. Carer. I acknowledge the thought. Greet it on the road like an acquaintance. Yes, that's what it means!

I am lying like a blind dopey old mole in the road waiting for the lorry to hit me. Somewhere deep in my moley consciousness I have an idea that when the lorry does hit me, I, the mole, will be able to deal with it. I wouldn't say I was moving at all. I wouldn't say I had a strategy. I only have the thought that I am two years older now since this all started and I haven't spent the entire two years lying in the road.

2.26

1 September 2010

Dear Friends

Here is some news. On September 4th it will be two years since my diagnosis.

A great deal has happened to us all in that time. My health has been generally good but in the last month I have started to have a lot of difficulties. My language is at times seriously impaired, impacting on my writing, reading and speaking. I struggle with these in many strange and peculiar ways.

My mobility has also become a real pain. This is due to the long-term effects of steroids. I move very slowly, especially up hills or stairs. But it is very good for me to see friends, and it helps me to converse when I do. I am not housebound at all, and go out for a bit every day but my energy fluctuates a lot. My chemotherapy is continuing.

I am still writing to some extent, though very slowly and mainly at night, and look forward to working. Marion holds us all together. Ev is flourishing, living with us and we with him.

Love

It is midnight. We have just got home and I carry Ev inert like a small sack in an anorak and put him to bed. Mentally I unravel the evening, spent round a table with friends who had not seen us for a while. I think of their unquiet eyes, their manner soft and alert to all the changes in us. We are such tricky guests: highly unusual. We demand all the attention in a given space. It is a huge effort and when alone, tiredness can roll into the vast, hollow space of me like a bank of fog. Sometimes when it's just the two of us I flicker off to vacancy in a click, to a kind of waking absence, blank and shallow breathing. Tom sits behind me very still under the lamp.

In this mode I am standing barefoot facing the mirror but not seeing my reflection when I hear my name said twice. God – what *is* that? My feet prick out with sweat as if a current has gone through them. I turn around, frightened. I don't understand this voice or where it comes from. Such a remote, far place, as if spoken in a chamber with all the furniture removed and the single word echoing and hollowed out hanging in the air. Here it comes again, not a word, an utterance. It is Tom's voice saying my name.

I have never heard my name like this, with so much mourning, and I will not hear it so again. I fold him to me. I understand it, its timbre, of course I do. He is losing my name. He is seeking it out as a word and feeling it on his tongue. How is it pronounced, this name? Irresolute now, he does not quite know it and in this speaking the whole shift between meaning and mechanism is breaking in on us. Everything follows from this I tell you. Everything. My name is a word like any other and though it means all of me to him, just like any other it may be lost. This is the trajectory of disease and if we think about it, it is a natural progression. But we do not think about it because disease is a wave and we are always, always in its wake. Like survivors floating behind we are knocked stupid. We must scavenge, pick things up and construct anew out of flotsam. A word that means my name can be lost just as well as a word that means door or coat or nail or boat. And we really do not grasp this. You'd think we might but we do not. There is no getting ahead of the wave and imagining our lives enough in advance to prepare, and maybe if we could, then we could not live as we do held tight and fast. We would simply drown, each alone and separate. Yet somehow, somehow, we still expect our sacred and familiar selves to be spared from oblivion until that endpoint when there is no more time left for us anyway. Marvellous. Miraculous. But why should that be so? In the last two days – two days! – we lose more in two days than you fail to recall in a year – all the names are going. We have been working through his essays on artists, running over the English lists. Tom has so much to say about them. He knows them still and their workings so well. But their names … Stubbs, Flaxman, Blake, Hooke … all going, all unspeakable. A new thing is voiced out of the chamber but this time a bit more distinct, soft and clear. *My boy,* he says. *I cannot say the name of my boy.*

2.27

On Box Hill we are exposed to all radiation, the bad and the benign. We are scoured and stabbed by leaves and blades of grass, by needles of rain and tiny stones. We endure it. We have come here willingly as we keep having ideas and one of them is termed The Outside. In my notebook are many overlapping lists and this one comes from the blunt, short-term list of things we want to do immediately, for pleasure. It is important to write down these ideas as otherwise the pressure on a given day can sometimes crush us and it is easy to forget that we ever had lives with interests and agendas. The effort, though, is great and it's no good ever trying to set effort against reward. Pleasure has to be won and all the better for it.

The little list has on it: Avebury, tick. Moro, tick. Plays known – the idea is that Tom, who loves and despairs of plays, having seen many badly staged – would comprehend and better enjoy a play he knew very well, no tick. Haircut, tick. Concert, tick. The concert was Lachenmann as David was playing in it. I drove Tom there and David and Martha brought him back and I savoured the normality of it through the evening like a long-lasting sweetie in my mouth. The Outside, tick, and so here we are on Box Hill.

The ground is chalky and poked through with tiny plants. In front of us is a vast view over some county, perhaps it is Surrey, and perhaps this is why people come here, but it is all is so far away as to register only as a zone of indistinction in a soft grey hue and I hardly know where I am much of the time. This is where you would come to watch the detonation of a bomb. It is a good vantage point to view a scale-less mushroom cloud easing into the sky over the whole region, displacing unimaginable volumes of air. After reaction, when knowledge touches atmosphere, there is no rescinding, only duration. I put my fingers over my eyes and imagine all the bones of my hands visible.

We have driven out with Heather and JK and they have a feast ready of chorizo and soft blanched cheese, green rocket, small pies and good tea in a flask. Heather walks Tom across the grass, past the holiday cabins that make up a little community like a survivalists' camp. It is abandoned. There are no survivors. We find a bench for Tom and the rest of us settle on the rug just as the rain begins. I know Ev loathes this. He hates extremes of weather grabbing at his arms and legs and roughing him about. I make myself as thin and hollow as possible and stuff him under my coat but he escapes to trail around forlorn in an adult anorak, his sleeves dragging on the ground like a wet ape. Tom is happy in his jacket and cap, sealed against the rain by exhaustion known only in dreams and the thrill of the high whipping clouds above our heads. But Ev is an instant complainant. Why should he endure along with us? Why indeed. I do not blame him but I am ruthless and I take no prisoners. I insist as long as I can. I insist and insist for just enough time to let me eat and then I give in. Back we go to the sealed car to warm it with our breath.

When the rain abates we venture out again to jump on a pile of gravel, kick a dead log and draw lines in chalk on the paving. No one else is around. Snails emerge. Ev finds a frisbee in the wet grass. All the while as we play we curl forward and back to Tom and around again, forward and back. Everywhere we go he is the context. He is with us in the heart of the game and outside it as a spectator and he watches it closely.

2.28

5 October 2010

Dear Friends

As some of you know already, Tom is in Guy's Hospital with a chest infection.

This is to tell you that he is likely to be there for at least another week.

He is in good spirits and we hope to keep them that way. To those who visited already over the weekend, much thanks. He had a wonderful and lively time.

Short visits are great if you can, as are cards, pictures, notes. Phone calls can sometimes work too.

Call me if you'd like more information.

Thanks as ever for your support.

With love

It is the dead, the straight dead of night and I have brought my subject and my object, the one who all this is about, into the hospital. He is wheezing. His face is florid and jowly, wrapped in a scarf and hat and his temperature has tripped over the killer number, 38. Thirty-eight means a phone call and immediate hospitalisation but we are OK. We are more than OK, we are delirious, in a high humour. It feels like a mad road trip, barking. A silky night-rain is falling as ever on the Elephant. Once out of the car we try one of the hospital wheelchairs but it's an abused thing, like a shopping trolley fit only for the bottom of the river. I can't unstick the brake, then I do, and I can't steer it, then I do, and now upstairs I can't push one side of the double door to get us into the ward where he is expected. We are unable to manoeuvre, dammed with all his weight listing to one side, and as I reverse for another assault I see the silhouette of the faraway nurse illumined through the glass like a Vermeer maid at the end of a quiet corridor reach down to press a button. I am through. Tom stretches the crook of his stick towards me as a falling man grabs for a branch and I pull him in after me just as the heavy doors move to close. His eyes have a full-on, wicked glaze. He is enjoying me going bum-ways in, laughing at the ridiculous, impenetrable doors that thwart the weak, at the deadness of the night and the great adventure of it all, another episode in our adventure of being and dying.

When the tests start up the nurses suddenly accelerate. I gauge the danger from their speed. This is serious. We should have come in earlier. Later we talk to the night doctor. He introduces me to her. *This is my friend.*

Ev says, *I have a sad feeling in my tummy because there is a problem.*

It is unanswerable. I rub his tummy.

I say, *When you have a sad feeling come and tell me and I will think of something to help. Talking is good, and hugs and rubs, but you know also, Ev, sometimes people are just sad.*

I am sad about Dad.

Me too. Let's go and see him in the hospital tonight and we will take the fishing game.

Tom has been in hospital for ten days now. We take in the fishing game and some sushi and we will have tea together. Sounds like a plan but it doesn't work out.

Here's the full weight of the thing coming down. The combination of Ev and Tom and the hospital is the one that doesn't work. I keep trying to get the peg to fit the hole but it doesn't. Too hard, too split, too wrong, so Ev hasn't been in since late last week. Today I have been in a meeting about Tom's work and Ev has spent the day with his cousins. He takes all of childhood as his due: mud, scooters, cars, cakes, sausages, the whole messed and mangled template scrumpled up and given to him like it was a normal everyday thing. When I come to pick him up I watch from the sidelines. He is hot, tired, happy, played out. Now it's time to visit the hospital. It is later than planned. Ev is more tired than planned.

Visiting hours look and feel the same. The same duo flank the bed of the man opposite. The Asian family are camped further down. Somehow, though I like this ward very much, I don't connect with the other patients, catch their eye or exchange pleasantries. It doesn't happen. Privacy is too lightly veiled. It's all too vital and too tender. In Poland I passed through a student hostel on a trip to Krakow and it was clear that the very young couple in the bunk opposite were on their honeymoon. They were on a tight budget. Rather than go out to eat, she unpacked the evening meal on the bed, a complex, elaborate thing from tins and packets: herring, pickles, eggs, Russian salad. The boy didn't lift a finger as she self-consciously served him on the lower bunk and they ate slowly as if in a restaurant under the eyes of the young Westerners who pretended not to look. So it is here.

Tom's voice is louder than usual. As his speaking becomes more difficult he can't control its volume so on the ward we are always broadcast with Ev carrying our noise still further. Ev is delighted to see Tom, and Tom him. This is the whole of my reward and it is a good one. They eat.

Tom has said that we don't have enough film of him and Ev. So I film. I do not eat. When the food is done I clear away and get out the fishing game. I film. I do not play. Ev doesn't know how to play this – or any – game and after a while Tom complains at the way he is playing. I tell him to stop. Tom now wants to do a bit of work on the laptop I have brought in. Ev wants to do a poo. This is an unhappy combination. Ev still likes to do his shit in a nappy. He is a boy of implacable habits and my feeling is that as his father is dying it is not the right time to try and shake them. Death and shit are joined enough without me forcing the issue. I figure that when he wants to change, he will. Trickier still though is that the ritual extends outwards; Ev likes a nappy, a chair to lean on, a book to read and he doesn't like being disturbed. He prefers to be in private with me in another room waiting for him to finish. But tonight he wants it differently. He doesn't want to go to the toilet. He wants to do it right here next to Tom on the ward.

We have a quiet little argument at high temperature and Ev and me go off to the toilet with a book. There is only one public toilet on this floor so we lock ourselves in. We may be a while.

Twenty minutes later my mood is vicious. I am still sitting on the floor staring at the walls and I have lost count of the number of people who have tried to enter by throwing their full weight against the door. No one tries the handle first. It is stifling. I want to be with Tom. Ev still reads his book. He hasn't done a poo. Visiting hours are nearly up. I roar at him quietly in the back of my throat, tearing the fibres of it a little. The choice is between roaring or full-on hysterics. I have to get out of here. Ev's colour is high. Lolling against the toilet he fiddles with the sanitary disposer and makes random conversation. Finally: *That's a good poo*, he says. There is nowhere to put the shitty nappy. It is too big to fit in the disposer so it goes in a bag in my satchel. Back we go on to the ward.

Tom is where we left him with the laptop. He is still copying down the passage he started with. Of course it would take ages, his handwriting is barely functional, but this long? I hadn't understood that he would want to work, having asked for Ev to come and see him. Why is he doing this? This is his child. It is late. Not the time not the hour. There is no time and no hour. He picks up what I am thinking and looks at me. *I still have more to do*, he says flatly. Ev starts crying. *I will copy it for you if you take Ev for a walk*. Ev cries flamboyantly and lies down on the floor of the ward. I smell shit in my bag. All the visitors have gone. The men are asleep or comatose. *This will take me two minutes. You must take him. Just take him and let me do this.* Tom tries but cannot shift him. Ev cries harder, piteous. I want to hit someone, either of them, both of them.

You are killing me, I say under my breath. *You are smashing me up and killing me. Leave then, don't visit.* There is never any choice. I cannot win. I know it. Death trumps; trumps me, the child, all our desires combined. *You should have brought him earlier,* says Tom. *He is too tired. Fuck you I was at a meeting sorting out your fucking life.* Ev is red-faced now and desperate, wailing. The cancer men grumble and toss in the blue light. Nurses look in our direction. They are right. What the hell is he doing here? I scrape and scrabble to get the words down. The pencil lead atomises in my fist. *Leave, leave.* He hisses. I find a pen and write down the line he wants underneath his seismographic hand.

Done. Done. Now, quick, everything in one move: bags, shoes, hat, computer, all done in one move done and let's get out of here. I wish I need never bring Ev here again. The two of them blow kisses. Tom stands static, a figure of solid, coalescing muteness. I think he would rather have his words and not us. Words will last, and we, well, we will do whatever we do. We are not creatures of posterity, we are too wayward, Ev especially. Ev points to a future somewhere else.

Walk us to the door, I whisper.

I want to go home, Ev whines.

Please, you must never, ever make me combine work with the child in this place. It cannot be done. I am carrying his poo in my bag. I have brought food for you. I have filmed you. You have no idea what it's like. You cannot imagine and you have no idea.

Leave. Just leave me.

I cannot, you know I cannot. I will not.

We blow kisses like normals. We move further off and blow some more through the two window panels in the door, the high one for me and the low for Ev. Ev does it for real and I in a kind of insensate storm.

Now that he knows he is leaving Ev changes tack. He is in high spirits and wants to get downstairs to see the automaton in the lobby of the nurse feeding the patient, though we rarely get the penny into her cup to activate her. We are too incompetent and slow on the roll so the patient never wakes to open his ghastly automaton mouth and take his medicine.

My throat feels burnt. After four goes we fail to get the penny in but Ev is cheered by the row of ambulances outside. At Elephant and Castle he asks *What is when you die*? I circle the Elephant in the dark. This is what I do. Circle the Elephant at night. *Die is to no longer be in this life with us. Die is to stop and be gone. We all have a life, Ev, and it is wonderful, many things happen and then one day it stops.*

By the time we are home he is asleep. Pity. I had wanted to offload a thousand apologies and cradle him and stroke his hair. Sorrow for my handling of it all, for my temper, for his father, for the disaster of our lives which sometimes flares and eclipses us but I cannot for he is asleep. For him this is best but for me, a great pity. I don't get to make my baby explanations and soften and soothe myself in doing so. Today we made a mistake. So instead of an apology I open a bottle of wine. If Tom had any wit he would text me right now. But he has not wit. Cancer is making off with his wit, his speech and his consciousness.

But yet, yet ... I take two thick swallows of red and text him. He calls back immediately. His voice is heavy but steady, still his own and to hear it is simply to be solved. To talk to each other is to have our medicine and to be remedied. How easy it is. We just open our mouths. I remember now. *We made a mistake*, I say. *Yes. We made a mistake.* He echoes me. *Sleep well. Sleep well. All love. All love. Till tomorrow.*

2.29

Tom is asking me to find a dressing gown and bring it in to hospital. This is how we do it.

It's a beautiful simple thing.

You have one.

And I have one.

Is it clothes?

Not really.

(He is a stickler for categories.)

Food?

No.

Bigger than a computer?

Yes.

It's very simple.

You like it and I like it.

(They are what we wear in the mornings.)

Do we use it in the kitchen?

Not really.

Many people have one!

It's just a simple thing.

I like it and you don't like it.

(He wants his second gown, the one I think is scruffy.)

When we finally get there – the blue, second-best dressing gown – I often pointlessly complain about one or more of his categorisations sending me off on the wrong track. He has a nice habit though, when you get something right and bring it in, or hit on the precise thought or word he is looking for, of saying, *Yes, that is perfect.*

Having an infection puts the brain further under pressure and impairs his speech heavily. There are certain stock phrases he uses with great tact and care in reference to the state of his thought. They change their nuances in different settings and over time you can work this out quite well: *This way and then another way. Never the case. Still a little bit.*

He refers to himself sometimes in the third person. He might refer to me as Ev or Tim or Jenny or whoever is in circulation. Green might be red. *One way but not the other way* tells me he can think clearly about something but not verbalise it. *In a different way* means he knows exactly what we are talking about in his head. About Ev he says, *He I can do – but the only one*, meaning he can say Ev's name aloud but no one else's. Ev's name can shift but today Ev stands for all names, the only one remaining. Tomorrow other names may return. A couple of times he says, *Ev – near that* and this means he is referring to me. The physically spatial applied abstractly is a construction he uses a lot.

Staying on top of these switchbacks is not possible and once when crossed a dirty, veiled look appeared direct from somewhere behind his eyes and he said coldly, *Well I shall say nothing at all then.* I see anger occasionally against me. But it never lasts. I don't know why not. What if I might be thwarting him? What if I might be not entirely on his side?

For God's sake, I am another human, I say. *I am not you, but another person, that's the problem.* He ignores this or simply can't afford to be conscious of it as he tasks me to execute his understanding and will in the moment that he wills it. Of course he does. I would. We all would. He would do everything himself if he could and the fact that he can't is merely an inconvenience.

For his own reasons Ev is also unforgiving of my autonomy. I ask Jenny.

Does Ev know I am human? It's driving me mad the way he uses my neck as a stair to climb on top of my head. The way he flings himself at me from the back of the sofa as I sit on it. He wants to smash me up. The lack of care I am finding really hard.

He is separating and he doesn't really like it, says Jenny.

But so aggressive!

Yes, so aggressive. Separating is hard.

I have disappeared out of range. I can hear things that others cannot. I can communicate with Tom and Ev but the conversation of almost everyone else is beyond understanding: squeaks and trills, a pipping, stuttering noise, high and without substance, like wind in old pipes. Are they talking about anything? It doesn't seem so.

2.30

One day this is what Ev will say.

Sometime in my third year my mother changed. She became a mad person. She looked after me OK, she was quite funny, but sometimes really angry, so angry that I would try to see if I could get her going though it was hard to work out why, as different things would set her off. She would scream and shout. It could be good but a bit scary. I would cry. Dad had a brain tumour, diabetes and he was very stiff. He couldn't really play much any more, he got his words muddled and sometime in that year he stopped being able to talk to me.

Tom is home again. I am in danger of doing Ev violence. I am a person in negative. I exist to facilitate the household. I have no more resources and though friends and family do what they can there is no support in the world that will make this work. Lack of sleep is eroding my mind. Tom falling away erodes it harder, right back to the cliff. The pattern is this. In the mornings at six when Ev wakes me, his brain starts applying its conflicting and irrational desires before mine has connected up my eyes. Waking is always a violent act. Until we are stabilised, this volatile period can be of any length and takes the form of a hazardous surge that builds, ebbs and flows but is shot through too with charmed clear stretches, through breakfast and on towards the magic hour between eight and nine when I have to get him out the door. This is the pattern unless something might happen to intervene, a small thing in itself maybe, a refusal, slowness, a silly thing that any three-year-old might do. And suddenly everything goes up. Wham. Explosion.

Today is the day I should return to work after the summer break and I am trying to get everyone ready. I don't recall the trigger but I can remember what follows because I watch it like a film, as if it is happening to someone else. I am beside myself. Melodrama doesn't cover it. I am unstoppable. I make a rasping, eerie sad noise that pains the back of my throat. I throw shoes downstairs, hurl Ev's clothes around, snap his toothbrush in half. The muscles of my face, legs and arms contract and my body seems to shrink by inches. I rush first outside in a mock leaving-the-house, slam the door, then charge right back in again to lie quivering on the bed upstairs. I cannot control my legs. I hear Ev howling in despair at the broken toothbrush. *Mend it, you broke it, mend it, Mummy, with tape.* I grip him and force his shoes on. I want to hurt him, I swear I do. I curse and beg and pray. It is ten to nine. It is not his fault. Nothing is his fault. Nothing is anyone's fault. What a pity. No one is to blame. Ev is not dressed. He has just got up yet his face is streaked with tears like a child's face at day's end. Tom has not got up. I must do Tom's insulin, test his blood sugar, make sure he has the rest of his pills, his breakfast, his probiotic drink, write instructions for the friend who is coming to sit with him while I am out, write instructions for the carers, get Ev to nursery, get myself to the chemist to sort out a wrong prescription, drive to work – can I drive? That's the start. Then when I am there, I must pay attention to what others say for six hours, come home, make supper and take us all up to north London on the first leg of a weekend away.

Today at nine none of this has happened. The world has separated out into constituent parts ever so gently and thirty minutes later I have not moved. I am still sitting on the front step with Ev. The street continues to look the same: terraced houses, brick and stucco in creams, greys and browns. My neighbour passes. I say *Hi* with my mouth shaped like a Hi. The eucalyptus opposite, pollarded last year, looks wrong as ever. The bins are still there like normal. A cat slides behind them. Yet I cannot rise or move from the step. My legs feel immensely long and delicate and my shins are like a faun's shins, thin and impossibly fragile. My ankles are made of china. I am soft and pliable as I handle Ev on my knee. Salt tears lap down my face on to my tongue, so strong and hot. He kisses me and I him. We are both waiting for something. We were in a terrible uproar and now it has stopped and we are looking at each other waiting to see what will happen next, as if someone else is going to decide. It really does not matter. We paw and squash each other. He looks beautiful. Did I dress him like that? When? A black jumper, drab cords, a light blue woolly hat jammed over his ears. I remember something. I remember he had stuffed himself under a chair, hands over his head and legs tucked in like a tortoise to get away from me. It was my son, hiding from me in terror.

So. This feels interesting, sitting here. I kiss him. This is what it feels like not to cope. Nice. I have come to land in a heap on the mat, my legs are tangled under me and I feel so much lighter and fresher. I am a faun, a Disney faun. I like it. I am giving up. Ev snuggles on to my lap. I will let it go. He wraps his hands around my neck. I will not take Ev to nursery. He climbs on my knee. I will not go to work. He strokes my sleeve. I will not sort out the drugs. He burrows in towards me smiling. My brain, in a storm, has tapped into a hidden reservoir of calm and found some deeply potent chemical. For the first time in a long while, I am stilled.

I had diamorphine once in hospital: oblivion as pre-warmed clouds borne by host angels. Though nowhere near as lavish, this has something of the luscious abandon, the overwhelming splash of the dose. No one is being managed. No one is coerced. No one is threatened. No one is going anywhere. Not Tom, not Ev, not me. Upstairs Tom eats his breakfast alone, drawn into himself for protection against my fury. It's a pragmatic position against rampant disorder, his response to uncontrolled response. I've seen him take it before. I cannot think about Tom now. He will be all right. This is what Ev needs. Me. And I need him.

Ian arrives as planned but I am bewitched in puddles of soft salts. I don't want this to stop and I am not confident of my body being vertical. Ev and I play like little bears, propping each other up and rolling over. Why did I not do this before? I have made a phone call apparently and now here is Roxy too. *Hello*. One of the carers arrives as well. *Hello*. He is a very elegant and beautiful Nigerian. I have never seen him before. I tell him there is nothing for him to do. Someone makes me a cup of tea *Thank You* and brings it to the step. It is the best tea. Someone takes Ev upstairs to play. Someone calls the nursery. Someone calls off work, for the day, the month, the term or beyond that even, I do not know.

2.31

The blue room glows turquoise in artificial light. There are many shades of blue in our living room, all mismatched against a single mustard curtain, the only thing I have ever had 'made up' in the old way. I took in another curtain as template and the man who took my order knew the date of the curtain I was copying and which factory produced it by the width of its deep pleat. It was an honour to mark the passing of such esoteric knowledge. I sit on the floor. The moon floats square in the window central to my vision. The room is restful. I am not watchful. I am not expecting trouble.

When Ev arrived home, arrived for the first time after being born, we brought him into this room and laid him on one of the sofas to look at him. He was asleep of course. After the hospital, the house smelled of decay: animal filth and chilled plaster, standing water, nameless fibres and the bodies of mites. Laying him down was like throwing a switch. Instantly he made a warm light around which to group. Simple. I can't remember what we did then, aside from look at him. Probably put the kettle on for tea. This was not so long ago.

Tom is writing at the table by the lamp. His speech is plausible again since he came home. He is back on the laptop. He is writing an article about a painting, Carpaccio's *St Augustine in His Study*: the saint turning to the window, the little dog following his gaze. He works carefully, like a jeweller, setting word beside word, revising, pausing to see how the words fall out and if meaning crawls into place. It is like casting runes. Written words or signs are guessed at and put into lines on a hunch with other, more known words and shuffled. His hunches are good. He knows exactly what he wants to say. Meaning catches up later. Or doesn't and the whole has to be reshuffled. Sometimes he will ask me to read something back or wonders aloud why a sentence is wrong. He gets stuck on *could* and *be*, but repeating these over a couple of minutes gets him to where *could be* makes multi-level sense in a click of context, spelling, syntax and meaning. It is very, very slow.

When printed, to the eye the text is absolute. You would not bother your head about its making. This is the first evening he has been able to write at all for a couple of days and being near while he works is so much my habit that I am lulled. We are both pleased he can type tonight. This morning he had said bluntly, *I cannot type*. I was blunt in return. *Then you will have to draw pictures*.

I pull the curtains. Winter! It is coming. We must lag everything with plastic, carpet the hall, draught-proof the windows, stop up the doors, wrap the boy in coats and make soup to last months. Will we survive it? We may not. I wonder why I feel content. The sum of our parts seems not ballast enough for the whole ship of trouble. But Tom under the lamp is doing his thing. Writing. This is the thing he loves to do. That he can do it still is breathtaking. His work is to make meaning and that it should take so much making only illuminates the endeavour. Like a spider spinning thread over yards or a bower bird bringing back stick after stick and knitting it together, the work has a goal. He does it beautifully even now. It is the miracle of consciousness and I am its witness. We are creatures. It is bliss.

2.32

25 October 2010

Dear Friends

If you have any free mornings, afternoons or evenings and would like to be a good companion/conversationalist/runner/supporter to Tom, then send me an email.

Many of you are doing such a lot for us already, don't feel you have to take on more, we are hugely grateful.

If you want to do this once, that's great, if you would like to do it on a regular or irregular basis let me know too. Fridays are already taken.

If I don't get back to you immediately don't worry. I'm trying to make some time off just for me and Ev to be together, and some time in the week for me.

We are going through a precarious, difficult but also strangely wonderful time. We are awaiting some drug news. We watch how things go.

With love

The home visit nurse is in our kitchen. She comes every now and then and generally has valuable and sensible things to say but here she says this to Tom. *On a scale of one to seven, how would you rate your quality of life?*

I am looking at his enormous legs and feet. The skin is so swollen and shiny that the flesh is not like flesh but more a sac that holds, that approximates a leg and the skin retains the imprint of a finger like memory foam. This is oedema, something that happens when the body stops functioning. He sits calmly at an angle to her, slightly absent, lightly bored, and says thoughtfully in his new voice, the muffled, internal one that he now uses. *That is a ridiculous question. Obviously on a daily basis we go – Oh God, Oh God, all the time at all the stuff to be done. But, generally, generally, it is wonderful. We are interested.*

My head jerks up, entranced. Even now with his duffed-up words he can nail the thing. Yes, we are interested.

One

Two

Three

Four

Five

Six

Seven

2.33

On Wingreen Hill Tom walks between two friends across the grass to the trig pillar. It is the highest point for miles and the air is forceful. From here Wiltshire spreads in a circular swirl like a hippy skirt of patches and braids in green and yellow with brown on the fringes as the season turns. Ev has just woken up and he is grieved at being pulled from the warm car into the wind. He is in a fury, pitiless. He will not walk and will not be carried. I am pitiless in turn, empathetic as stone. I will him to be quiet, spit threats and tiny curses into his ear and press him close against me under my coat, trying to shelter him, stifle him and muffle him out. This is the end of walking. All our situations now, however banal, come near to collapse. Ev the little white demon gathers all his strength to burn hotter and stronger than me and as we are in company I cannot just kill him and bury his body. I want to take a photograph. He will not let up his spasmic screaming. *Please just let me take a photograph*. I do it, one click, two, then abandon. We return to the car.

The car placates him instantly. He knows he has won and we watch the three tiny figures, his dad flanked by two others moving away from us across the grass towards the copse and towards the horizon. If only Tom could continue and just keep walking, away from all this. That would be something. I would urge him on even though it would be to lose him. What will be left of us? What fragments will we pull together in this wind? Mercy, well there is none. *It is the linear thing I really object to, Ev*, I say, *the unfolding of a set trajectory. We are all knowledge and no power.* Ev has a biscuit in one hand and a drink in the other and he kicks his boots happily against the back of the seat. He likes being here with me. The wind continues to howl but in the car we are cocooned and the rest is happening far off as if on a screen.

I look at the photograph I have taken. Tom is a wrapped figure leaning just off true. He is a spaceman. He is not in the world. The image is an inversion. I see only a small part, the part pertaining to the photograph. He sees the whole of it and me in it.

2.34

One at the bottom, one at the top and another one in the middle, then a one along up the side. Ev is writing the letter E on the blackboard. He has seen a little e and says it is wrong. *This is how it should go*. The sun is immaculate in an autumn sky. It's been a rough day so far. I have been crying a whole lot. It's three o'clock and we are not yet out of the house.

The size of the tumour means that Tom wears his glasses at a 40 degree angle. He can put them on himself with his left hand and they sit at a rakish diagonal on his face. I am surprised they stay on but they do. It is functional and comical. Everything is perfectly natural. The angle of the spectacles is an optimal one, as if all along his glasses have been working towards it. I have a photo of him, glasses askew, leaning forward to look at a book. He looks like a creature lunging on food. Now he is studying the room. *I like all these things*, he says, waving at the CDs. *And I like all these things here*. He seems in awe, his voice soft as he looks around gesturing to point all of it out. I follow his gaze. *It is beautiful ... the beautiful thing down here ...*

We are surrounded by our possessions. I am surprised that things remain where they are without agency. Nothing would ever move unless I picked it up or kicked it. I do not clean anything and I tidy very little. The balls of dust are now of a size that Ev uses them as puffs of smoke and sticks them on the funnels of his trains with Blu-tac. The number of objects in a single home is incredible. I am as astonished as he is. We think we are not materialistic but we have a child and we value things in relative and unstructured ways: vast numbers of books, piles of toy cars, CDs, assorted objects, bits of paper, unidentifiable pieces of stuff, all waiting for us to move them, use them, deal with them. Just to notice them would be a benediction. As they no longer matter I have stopped seeing them until he brings them to my attention. But I understand his enjoyment. He values the opaque and solid rummage of our lives. These are our familiars. He is waking them all up. Gifting them with a look.

I have just realised that Tom can no longer get into the shower unaided. While I help him do this and wash his hair I treat it as an anomalous fact, something curious to note but kept at a distance as if it doesn't really concern me. If he cannot do it now he will do it even less well later. I focus on the shampoo and keeping my hands busy, though inside I can feel something else going on and the implications for us and for our life are working their way through my soft tissue like a worm through earth. The worm has a hard head and a cold tail. In Nigeria as a child I got a parasite in the sole of my foot. I watched it generate its white track and plough out a pattern like a microscopic intestine beneath the skin before my mother stabbed its body with a needle and picked it out bit by bit. Getting Tom dressed takes a further while. But we do get there finally, out into the sunshine.

I drive metres up the road to the car park to find the one disabled bay. It is blocked. Again it takes a while but sometime later everything is accomplished though it is now nearly the end of day. We are parked and the path stretches level ahead and looks walkable even by him. I wouldn't mind some silence, just to walk together, but Tom is unstoppable. Language is pouring out in his cracked pot and glue vocabulary. He is on witty form and gets into a monologue of chatty explanations and comments, pitted with caustic humour and surprise observations all fuelled by the desire to converse. A friend has just been visiting him at home and on the path he mimes him for me, gurning his stricken face moaning and sorrowing at his condition in the style of a Japanese *Noh* player. *Poor G*, he says, *I told him, 'But it is wonderful.'*

He makes me laugh. He sounds so happy and this is infectious so I start to be so too. I feel my spine lengthening. My neck moves fractionally out of lock. We link arms.

I can't do this in one way, but in a different way I can, it is all exactly the same. I have heard this a lot recently but now I attend to it very closely.

You mean that maybe you can't say a word but in your head you can.

YES.

You mean that all the vocabulary that was available to you before is still available in your mind, just that you cannot speak it, or only a tiny fraction of it.

YES!

But poems, songs, the lost ones, are they there even now?

NO. No, I cannot do them, or just a little.

I am still. His tone is so confident, its confidence laced with patience, courteous and self-deprecating. *I am so lazy*, he always said. Tom's natural good manners are set to maximum nowadays, as if aware that a person who cannot really speak must gather all his charm in doing human work with other humans. Speech needs exquisite care not to waste a drop or syllable. I adore this strength, the determination to let me know what is and exactly how it is. The humour in his voice is undiminished. It fizzes through his words like soda. Illness has left his character simply intact. A hurricane can destroy everything but leave a single house, its walls, roof, doors, windows standing and not a curtain gone. An improviser like him could live in it still.

On the hill the trees are in silhouette against the sun. The light is fond of us and comes in low. Suddenly I have a thought.

When you cannot speak at all, Tom, you will still have yourself and all your reserves of brain and consciousness for company and because you are you and I know what that means, I know that you will have the whole world inside and you will be perfectly all right.

YES! EGGSAAACTLY.

So that is what you mean when you say that it is amazing and wonderful.

YES.

YES!

Shadows are gone. The sun is gone. The park is emptying. Just us.

You know, in all this crap and running about and managing this cancer, we must keep doing this, this conversation, keep checking in with each other because now I can think again. It's like a clear space that I can reach. It makes me remember how much I trust you. Because I know you, so of course it makes sense. Sometimes in the deluge of what needs to be done I forget and now I feel better, so much better. This is the way, the only way that we can go on together. We must remember.

YES!

Well, just so you know how things go, and how the things that go, go. We walked this walk on Monday. On Tuesday we heard they would fund the new drug, Avastin, and his right side started to fail. On Wednesday we walked a tiny distance, less than 15m, to a restaurant to celebrate the news and nearly couldn't make it. On Thursday we stayed at home and on Friday we stayed at home again and he couldn't walk to the kitchen so we brought the table into the living room. On Saturday he couldn't walk to the toilet and four people walked him out of the house and down twenty-three of the thirty-eight steps to the ground, into the car and into hospital.

2.35

Ev's favourite outing is the Imperial War Museum. There are some understandable reasons for this and others I find more obscure. But the depth of his love for *Imperial* as he calls it is intense. He tags its suffix on to other museums he likes, Natural War Museum, Science War Museum, Horniman War Museum as if to annex them to his desire. It is his first joke. Heavy hardware, guns, planes, rockets and giant trucks – it all makes sense for a boy his age although at home his games seldom focus on battle and involve a multitude of operations. Maybe it is the word itself he finds unfathomable. God knows what children think of it. Boys love to hear the plosive sound aloud. It seems to distil into one syllable all the focus and energy of staring into a fire.

Today I have brought him here in despair as he is fractious at home and the museum is an easy bus ride away. Tom is in the house working and Andy is his companion. They are happy and settled and Ev is one too many. I am not mentally equipped for an outing. The only bits of the museum I can stand are the 1940s house and the replica section of submarine. I walk around the rest in restless jabbing motion as a pigeon moves, staring at the ground. My attention span is near zero.

Even so I notice something new. On a low plinth in front of me is a piece by Jeremy Deller, *Baghdad, 5 March 2007*. It is the mangled wreck of a car hit by a bomb and it brings across the world, in the way that artists do, one of the cars that was parked on Mutanabbi Street that day and sets it down here. Thirty-eight people died in the explosion. This is an act of transportation: things that are far come near. I did not grow up in the kind of Christian religion that believes in transubstantiation, very much its opposite, yet strangely this I could almost believe in, the idea that something can be something else, that matter can be perfectly and exactly two states in the same moment, body and blood. I cannot read the texts and can barely comprehend what any of the objects in plain sight are for, let alone grasp this ontological complexity. But I look at it, intense and puzzled, until Ev grabs my hand. He wants to go to the submarine.

We are in the submarine when I get the news about Avastin. The displays in the sub haven't worked for a while. The crew die every time because the pressure gauges are broken and the undersea audio is stuck on whale noise. My expectations are low. I follow Ev around and my aim is to keep him in sight and get through the afternoon. His capacity to explore his environment with the barest input from me is still impressive. The exhibit is a narrow space, very popular with young children, and I get the text as Ev is flirting with another child on the narrow submariner's cot by flicking the curtains of her bunk.

FUNDING FOR AVASTIN APPROVED.

My breath leaves my body and I step back hard into another parent. What is this? A litany of disjunction: public/personal, home/world, child/father, death/death deferred. It is all explosions and aftershocks. There is the trauma of love and there is the trauma of death but ultimately it is all trauma. Only oblivion will make it stop. A howl sits in my throat. I wish I could change places with this other parent, the man I have just hit. He is a French dad on a museum trip to London with his child. I wish I were him.

The submarine is too confined for this news. There is no air. Ev's game is up and I drag him into the wider space overlooked by heavy artillery. At home Tom and Andy are in high excitement and the commotion in my head reaches a thrill. This news may mean something or nothing but it is the one thing that is left to do. We have always done the next thing and the next thing and the next thing and this is the last thing. Someone has thought it worth a try. It is a call to action so of course we take it. The way is not barred.

2.36

Later and later people come to our house: Laura or Tim or Tom or Jenny, Roger or Charles or Richard or Mark. I have been up for so long I go to bed, leaving them at it below. But I listen. I want to be party to it by proxy. Tom's clothy tongue is infused with humour. *Dad's voice sounds like Santa*. This is how it goes – intense pauses, jams, prompts, small running grooves, electric bursts and ruffles of talk spilling over each other. Sudden claps of laughter. They are intoxicated. Nobody is keeping quiet. What are they talking about? The things that matter to them: memories, arguments, positions. They are going over the territory they are going to lose. For Tom the later it is the better he speaks. Fluency comes with darkness.

Ev sleeps like the dead. I lie like them, attentive to the voices on the black stairs. I am a stone-carved tomb-wife sealing the bed with my long back. What are they talking about now? Not sure. Drifting. When I lay in bed as a child listening to adults talk below, I thought that this was the only talk that mattered. It's the same excitement. This is the only talk that matters.

The next day is the first in so long that Tom has pain. We are not sure what to do. After each operation he was given some standard painkillers but as soon as he could express a view he declined them. I have taken more painkillers than him. The brain is an unfeeling lumpen thing, a blockhead. It does not hurt. But now here it is. Pain.

He tries to describe it to me, but our capacity to comprehend another's hurt in the place where it hurts is very poor so I have little idea what it feels like. Visually it looks like a headache roving just in front of the scar-place and behind the eyes. I am worried about his eyes. They look to be next in line for attack.

I have lost track of the drugs: Epilim, dexamethasone, omeprazole, metformin, mesalazine, clobozam, frusemide, alendronic acid. I want Tom to eat a bit of food before he has a painkiller. Many of them say

Take with food. But drugs are the opposite of meals.

I stand behind him stroking his back as he spoons cornflakes slowly into his mouth. A little milk drips down his front. Ev joins us. *Me too*, he says in a whiny voice. I pour him some cornflakes and he sits at a companionable right angle next to Tom. *What about me*? I start to stroke his back too. We make a tableau vivant in which I am wholly emblem, like an inn sign or tarot card: *Woman stroking two backs*. Content, he spoons cornflakes slowly into his mouth. A little milk drips down his front. For a long time I move my hands in circles while I stare out of the window at the trees.

2.37

It is early in the morning, only 8 a.m., but the disaster has already happened, pitching me from sleep blankness into deep blackness, and I am gathering myself post-wave. Are all mornings like this? Maybe. I can't tell. Some ground has been reached. I am no longer scrambling to catch things as they fall, not running or pleading, just sitting.

I grip a cup of coffee. Ev has had his breakfast. Tom has had his drugs and is in place on the sofa. His body in this position is doubled in size, armatured and buttressed by all the pillows from the sofa opposite, now just a nude frame, its dirt exposed. He sits like a giant surrounded, commandeering the room, pronouncing and gesturing, but quite often sleeping. Every one of these last six days I have watched something fall away. This is collapse. He cannot rise or walk on his own and I can see the end of this last phase, the attempt at being a family at home, slipping away as the last of night turns into morning.

At 6 a.m. the dark floor was pooled with piss. Everything happens for the first time and then you know and the knowledge after that is never surprising again. So it was here.

Ev comes in flying at high altitude. In full flow he moves from room to room, his voice mobile, never halting, rising and falling in a kind of song packed with overlapping narratives half-heard and strung together and shunted along by their own weight. The jet in his hand is cruising at shoulder height and he keeps it at a careful, even distance to the floor. Ev knows about sonar and radar and the vocabulary of destruction. He speaks the death language. The jet and three Lego trains are the subject of the commentary. The action derives from *Godzilla* and the impending disaster is noisy and happens in real time. In contrast to the madness of the last two hours this is translating as normal. Out of habit I say *Shhh, quieter*. *It's all right,* says Tom. *Good.*

Usually I feel that Tom cannot perceive Ev in full play mode. He is like a musical score with too much going on, some crazy nineteenth-century Romantic music, the full orchestra and chorus. Tom rejects these now. Mahler has gone. I didn't like him anyway. But I notice other musics going too. Tom needs a purer line to follow. The music may be complicated but the sound should be a single or double-actioned thread with no lyrics: Bach, Rameau, Couperin, Debussy. Bach in fact. Bach is where we are at the moment.

Look, Mum, says Ev, *here are the buffers and then this jet just comes like this and it burns the city but not the trains they go in the water they are safe the water will not burn this is concorde Mum look this is concorde Mum Mum it makes a really big noise heeeere it comes and the trains are clever they are safe neeeearghhnaaaaww, crassshhh, nothing will hurt the trains the fire trucks will come and kindly put water on the city and here come the Japanese people there is an explosion but the trains are in the water already so they are safe neeeearghhnaaaaww.*

The sofa is raised 30 cm and we sit overlooking the bay with the boy and the trains and the fire trucks. The extra height twists the sofa's function beyond itself and turns it into a shelf or ledge. I like it here. As long as nothing else bad happens this is the place where me and Tom and Ev are just about OK. If I lean back I can dangle my legs like a girl in the sun on a pier. It is sweet for me, less so for Tom for whom the sofa serves as everything: bed, seat and refuge. The hospital bed has not arrived and will not do so until our paperwork moves through the encoded triple-tiers of Social Services. What would we do with a hospital bed when it got here anyway? And where would we put the three existing sofas? We love each equally and their functions have high value. The black and green for me, the old pink one for him and the shabby blue for the boy. Our whole life takes place now on the pink and the three of us are often found on it. The hospital bed if it arrives will be functional but have no value. It will be here for the duration and then it will leave. Yes. The duration.

I have one arm around Tom's shoulder. The other hand curves over my coffee holding it safe and the light is building fast. We are facing directly towards the window. We are both ready. Here it comes. *Heeeeeeere it comes.* The sun suddenly spills over the roof opposite and crashes like a cymbal into the tree outside in a smash of liquid and solid light. The tree, a False Acacia Aurea, and the sight of it crowding the window was why I wanted the house when I first saw it. Oval pinnates of yellow-lime illumination frill and burst at the glass and reflect glory on us inside. We are gaudy with the stuff, dressed and dazzled. I am suddenly at peace. Where does this feeling come from? It is because we are together in our rightful place, in and around each other. This is *our* disaster. There can be no other name to give it. Ev's jet is mended around its middle with tape. It has lost its noise so Ev does it manually. He lands it on Tom's stomach. *Craaasssshh. Neeeearghhnaaaaww.* It lifts off again and wings away, banking sharply. He circles and returns, transferring the jet now to the other hand to stroke Tom with his free hand on the mound of his middle. Ev looks up at us. His eyes are wide, he is exultant: at us, the place, the jet, the light. I must take a photograph. I do not move. What will I remember? What will he remember? This feels gorgeous, voluptuous, yet Tom is leaving us now, really leaving us. *Beautiful* says Tom.

The blue room moves into its highest phase. As the early sun strengthens and the saturation of the walls grows towards maximum, these light levels are what its colour is for. In all other circumstances I refute fate. I do not believe, but here is the one instance. Out of all the permutations on the colour chart, I chose this blue.

Two hours later I make a phone call and we take Tom into hospital. I couldn't have told you in advance that I was going to do this but with Tom asleep and Ev at a neighbour's, I make a judgement. Once fixed on it is immediately executed. I don't know how. Everything I do is gilded by the aura of gold leaves. It is a Saturday but all external operators are somehow in place to make it work. I phone Dr B. She phones me back.

Dr B phones the Registrar. The Registrar is on call on the ward. The Registrar phones me back. The bed is free. To have the bed we must get there and claim it. Here is a catalyst for action. Its momentum unfurls joy in both of us. Though Tom can barely walk, the project is urgently to leave the house and we must not fail. Failure means the task will be given over to others. Tom will become the object of someone else's day, an ambulance job or a problem to be slotted in. He will become work and we will have to wait. Because he is ours, he is not a problem and he is not work. We will not wait. We just need to find a way to do it.

I call Tim, who comes immediately, and then the doorbell rings and there stand two more unbidden. We are a team. The four of us help him down the stairs. Tim behind, the Faller-back and Matt on one side, the Leaner. On the other, Marianne the Mover to work the foot and I in front am Cantor, Caller, Way-clearer and Cheerer. *Just keep coming, keep coming to me, that's it, wonderful.*

I can see that Tom's right foot does not belong. It has become a felt-shod object to be shifted by hand. He can no longer do it. The right hand is wavering too, wavering and waving, it gently sifts the air, uncertain of its status. The brain is losing agency over the right side. It has limited traction and pull and can no longer assert itself. All this is visible but what is also visible is that we four are only manual operators. It is Tom who is doing the work. The body will not move without the brain and Tom is the brain. He is highly concentrated and exquisitely slow. A distilled essence of himself, an incredible, crystalline-thinking, new-made self has been forced into being. He thinks himself down the stairs.

Transparent sheets of consciousness like the thinnest filo or gold-leaf layers gently rub against each other, crumble and become dust. I cannot take my eyes off him. He is mustering all remaining power over his body stair by stair. The whole empire is falling. It is spectacular, unbelievable. My eyes doubt but persist. I will see it. A cortège of one and three descending. The man in the centre, the one behind and two at the side form an awkward crowd tight-knotted on the stairs as if jammed into a narrow painting. Thirteen black stairs, a turn, the bookcase on the left, a narrowing, three more stairs unpainted and wooden. Then a long stretch of flat, past pushchair and scooter, six more stairs, stone now and we are in the autumn air. The foot hesitates. Down the kerb to the car. A shuffle of yellow leaves. So a man leaves his home.

SECTION 3

3.1

1 November 2010

Dear Friends

There are two pieces of news. The first is that Tom is in Guy's Hospital as of this weekend. His mobility on the right side deteriorated sharply last week and it is no longer wise for him to be at home.

He is in very good spirits and we hope to keep them that way. Visits are a pleasure for him. He is in the same ward as before. Cards, pictures, notes are very welcome. Phone calls can sometimes work too.

The second news is that funding for him to receive the chemo drug Avastin has been approved. We heard this last week,

> and are delighted and surprised. This is scheduled to start on Wednesday.
>
> It's a very extreme time, deeply precarious, but also amazing. Tom has been doing a great deal of talking and writing lately with the help of friends.
>
> All our love

On the eighth floor we are somewhere else entirely. The high tower creates artificial currents that storm around its base but the fast lift shoots up and at the top the air is tamed. On the ward our breath mixes closely with the breath of others. The temperature is constant but coming in from the outside I never get it right; too many clothes, too few. In this anodyne place, sealed tight, perversely Tom is become a sensualist, a volupt of the flesh. He seems to have lost his edges, or they have loosened and settled and I am unsure quite where they now lie. Since coming in, he has lost too the ability to move unaided, yet though he is so fiercely embodied, and in a body that does not move, a body that is now a serious problem, he is in a strange way, blooming.

He always had a great deal to say about being embodied. In art primarily. *Being a figure in a picture, what's it like?* He identified closely with the pressures of embodiment, its expressiveness, the extraordinary business of representation. The very otherness of the physical self as it is becoming is of interest to him. The fact that it is *his* makes it no less interesting.

Physically he has much to learn and do, for novelty renders everything unstable and there are endless repercussions to not comprehending your own foot, but mentally, here is the new world and he is hard at it. He can move only with the agency of others. Not like an object or thing, a dog in a sack, a man in a sleeping bag, but like a potentate, an oligarch, an exotic entity. As the trappings of this state are prosaic – hoist, blanket, straps, chair – I cannot help feeling that this is mighty clever and that it requires a double-act of acute skill on his part and on the part of his nurse-attendants: him to demand it and them to give it. He has no physical embarrassment. No shame. Because this registers as absence, the importance of it might be overlooked but I have come to value its impact greatly. It is not dissimulation, just something played completely straight, ideological and lightly worn. This is not a moral issue. It is his body going wrong. Illness gets coated like mucus with physical shame. The absence of shame is enlightening. There is nothing standing in the way.

We have by far the best spot on the ward for a person who has no interest in being left in peace, the first bay after the entrance, next to the nurses' station with a window on all their doings. Mounted on a herd of wheelie chairs squeaking and rubbing, the nurses chat, confer and sit on the phone for hours. They tick off lists while kicking their legs and sometimes sail abruptly over the lino to expedite whatever it is they are doing without getting up. Around the ward they move fast but without noise, like ushers or people who have studied Alexander Technique. Is this in their training? How to move? Like dancers they carry their personality in their bodies and like dancers the variety of their bodies adds colour to their skill: benign, tense, calm, funny, hassled, smooth, spiky, serene; it's a volatile mix. This is our environment. He is raw here, as alive as ever and more demanding: more and more.

Looped over the nightlight above his bed, so visible at all times, is a sign in paint on board, a work by Bob and Roberta Smith that arrived in the post. It reads I BELIEVE IN TOM LUBBOCK. On the back, unseen, in red scrawl is the further message, *The best drugs are visual*.

Around the bed the paper curtains are a thick lapis blue. They limit our space to a few square metres yet make a condensed theatrical setting in which everything he does has exaggerated impact, sending waves crashing on to his audience. This can be comic, entertaining, or alarming depending on your mood and the closeness of your friendship. Eating a piece of salami, being understood, having his head stroked, drinking a coffee, watching a film, hearing an anecdote, hitting on a word, listening to music, seeing a friend come round the corner: these are raucous pleasures and his response is deep and sexy. *EGGSAAACTLY* he will drawl, eyes wide on full aperture and radiating on the object of his attention.

The food is shocking, worse beyond jokes. I get a knot in my stomach every time it comes round. *I am being beaten here*. To be sure I am not exaggerating, I try eating it: one day, gristle in sauce, on another, cold, diced, par-cooked turnip and carrot medley. This is not what we eat. This is not what anyone should eat, sick or well. If I had strength for a fight, I would fight. As it is, I feed him: paella, pasta, salad, soup, sausage, sushi, sometimes from home or from the market. Though I, and many of our friends, do our utmost to offset the demoralising effect of bad food, I cannot orchestrate three meals a day and at times he has to knuckle down. Drugs have sent his appetite through the roof. Lots of rich snacks are coming in and he would eat all day, unchecked. It takes me a while to realise that this is what he is doing.

Running counter to the expansion of his personal realm, his senses are being neatly eroded by the environment so that when anything novel does penetrate it is with the force of an explosion like a Chinese firework in a narrow alley. Smell, sight, taste, are being muffled and tamped down by cotton sheets, poor meals and rows of sick men in pale gowns and trousers. I push him out in the wheelchair down to the river, pitting my strength against the streaming pedestrian flow at London Bridge, past the occult, half-built, half-dead-already Shard, its glass splinter at exactly half height. It is Babylon. The builders, commuters, the smokers and sellers, are swift and toxic. The experience of being outside is hugely tiring, more than I grasp till later, but he is amazed and energised. He loves it. It is a brutal intimacy. In a wheelchair you are not up at people's faces but stuck around the waistline, the trunks and torsos, the hot seams around arms and legs where material tucks and sits and sweats and doesn't fit. God how they stink, their fags, their clothes, the food they eat as they walk! His senses are being forced by the hospital regime on to an ever-retreating baseline and back on the ward, a spoonful of a mild Thai dish from the market – a treat, I thought – sends his colour rocketing, and he needs ten minutes of groaning and drinking water to recover. Stilton on an oatcake brings on an opera of sighs. He nearly weeps.

Demands are multiplying. Today I must bring in a Barbour jacket, a blanket, pomegranate juice, an orange and a banana, nail scissors and a certain straight-sided mug. The jacket and the blanket are in readiness for an outing. Three of the five versions of Cézanne's *The Card Players* have been brought together in an exhibition at the Courtauld and we have long had a plan to see it. This is a proper trip with complex logistics. It means mobilising Sacha and Vivien, a wheelchair, transport and an afternoon for the project. I learn so much that I previously did not know about the world of the immobile that it is hard to believe it all takes place over a few hours. At random: I learn about the casual indifference of the London cabbie to the wheelchair user and that the clearance on accessible entrances is measured in millimetres less than a knuckle. I learn how intractable it is to push a grown man around for hours and how spontaneity is the privilege of the able-bodied. In solid counterpart to all this grief, I learn about the lengths nurses are prepared to go to assist a purely recreational and ambitious project by one of their patients.

In the gallery the works are drawn inward. The display is as concentrated as its subject. Cézanne's farm workers hunch like Easter Island statues: the one from the Met, the one from the Courtauld, the one from the Musée d'Orsay and a clutch of other canvases. We have a long hour.

Tom says, *You must do it*. This means he can't initiate the conversation but if I begin, he can join in. I move into mode beside the chair with our friends as outriders and we go slowly from painting to painting and back and forth between them. I am not so ready. I hate these

Cézanne figures, their deaf-blind maleness. We get into a small dispute about chronology. Tom turns out to be right. A painting is such a complex thing however you describe it: a made object representing something else, a painted surface on board or canvas, an illusion, a formulation about the world, a sign that stands for itself, a historical event, a moment in a series. How do you stop looking when you know that your looking is finite? When have you looked enough?

We are already late. Tom is exhausted with the effort and he starts to shiver. Trying to get him home in the evening rain I stand on a traffic island in the Strand signalling for a taxi. The one-way system means a cab must make a tricky manoeuvre to reach him. I tell the first cabbie he is to pick up a wheelchair. *OK, Lady,* he says, and I watch his tail lights blend with the traffic streaming in the other direction. No one else is stopping. The slanting rain is freighted with ice. London rain in winter is pure sorrow. Will I ever be sad in a normal way again? I look forward to that. Finally I flag down another and get in myself, forcing him to make the turn. In the middle of these hostilities, a lady from a hospice agency calls me. She is phoning to tell me that as a carer I am eligible for complementary therapy, massage, acupuncture and aromatherapy sessions. Manically cursing I shout expletives at her down the phone.

3.2

Tom wants a book. We talk on the phone. *The oyster* he says. *No. Damn. OK where is it? In my book. Try again … The oyster, no, Oster.* I know he doesn't want to read Paul Auster. *Let's try by elimination, is it on your desk?* We are not getting anywhere ... *Let's leave it ten minutes, Tom, and you'll get it. I'll phone back.*

A short time later I get a phone call. *The-Eng-Lish-Au-Den. Yes, good, where? The poetry shelves in the bedroom, a pink and white book.* Here it is, *The English Auden*, collected prose and poetry, sitting like a miracle. *And a Fessarus.* That's easy, Roget's. We get there. So far we always get there. Each time we do this I try to think of it as a puzzle to be solved so it doesn't hurt me.

Later, I will find this whole conversation – *the english auden on the poetry shelves, in our bedroom, pink and white, collected prose and poetry* – written in crabbed pencil in one of his notebooks. Tom is a notebook user of long standing. He uses them for writing and drawing and has one on him at all times. It's a sight I have grown fond of: notebook held high and settled comfy on the chest, pencil in hand, a sideways look as if something really *was* just over there, and then a sudden light scrabble, a scratch of lines marking the relay of a thought into a word. The habit of reaching for a notebook is an action similar to smoking, or how smoking used to be, urge rolling into action wherever the need surfaced. Over the last months his notebook use has gone viral; their role is wildly varied and their function starker. Writing everything down on the spot is a necessity. It is not simply a question of memory. The word may not be his to write later. There is nothing that does not need a notebook. They mark the continuation of his existence.

I find them in every room at home: tiny, black books, unruled and soft with very few words to a page, sometimes only one or a single drawn shape formation. He was always profligate with paper. His handwriting was so terrible that I can't quite tell if it is much worse now. He uses propelling pencils of a kind I cannot master. I don't know why, I am not clumsy but I have never learned to handle these. The leads are the narrowest gauge graphite, like spider web hardened with spit. His touch must be so light.

After the first short stay in hospital in August when his drugs soared from two to eight a day, I took up my own notebook. Its black cover warms the length of my hand in my pocket and it goes with me wherever I go. At the front is Tom and his needs: medication, words spelt out between us, what doctor X said, what doctor Y said, diagnoses, dates of fits, questions needing to be asked, phone numbers of professionals. At the back, taking up far, far fewer pages are lists of tasks that aren't directly to do with cancer. The front overran the rear a while ago but the book remains so current that I stick an identical one on to its cover with Sellotape and continue.

Now he phones for something else: *There are three of them, white yoghurts*, he says. *No, you can't want three white yoghurts. No, I know, but I want the biggest ones you can find. Yoghurts. No, sweet, still not making sense. OK.* A short time later he calls back: *T–shirts. Yes, I know.* I had guessed already. They are packed. So it goes.

When we are face to face we can do this readily. On the phone we speak across terrain like a quarry: great chunks of rock smashed to rubble, a landscape of boulders, incoherence, dust and vertiginous slide broken by small, un-signposted passages of narrowly traversable rock along which we meet. Every conversation has to navigate a different route and we cannot ever learn a path and use it again. Except when we can. The true thing is that nothing holds true always. Suddenly, we will have a phone call, usually late at night, and it will be just like what you might call old times except they are recent and continuous times. A perfectly beautiful verbal pearl about nothing, socks or sleep, but an incandescent bubble, a capsule of connecting light. If I had a belief in agency behind all this I might complain that this is cruel. As it is, I do not have that luxury.

I am a tiny diver seen from the ground black against the sun. I am on the highest level of the tower. My approach is good. I have paced myself, jumped and bounced twice, taking up all the energy of the board into my body and I am on the rise. It is a perfect takeoff. I feel a warm exhalation of breath rising from the ground willing me on. Except that my elevation continues. It does not stop. Velocity is taking me up too far, surely I must go into the curve and fall of the dive. Mentally I am ready for descent. Gravity drags on my thighs. The weight of my head, the heavy, so troublesome head, should weigh me down and slow my ascent, but still my rise continues. I hear my friends call out in alarm. The high-diver goes up, arcs, controls the turn and cuts the water silently without ripple or bleed, vertical as a plumb line with the head as lead. These are the rules and gravity is the agent. I am slowing, ready for the turn but it does not come. I am slowing, not rising, not turning, not falling. What is to happen? Surely I will stop, I will hang in the air and never fall. But no, even the stop does not come. Nothing comes but upward movement, held now to an imperceptible float. I am still moving, way out of reach, but my mind is thinking only of the turn and my body is poised to plunge to earth.

3.3

5 November 2010

Dear friends, dear colleagues

Tom has written a long piece about his life and work since being diagnosed with a brain tumour in 2008.

It will appear in the Observer this Sunday – 7 November 2010.

We thought you would like to read it.

For those of you who are far away, it will also be online.

Feel free to pass this message on to other friends, readers, supporters of Tom.

A case conference has been called to decide the future. In my mind I run the future forward and back all the time so I wonder if they could possibly have more ideas about it than I do. In advance of this meeting I am uneasy and prepare for it as you might before a performance. I go on the Internet.

I am looking for another home. It is clear that ours will not work any more. At the top of the search after putting in my key words – local area, ground floor, one-person, accessible – I see something so singular and fitting that I don't quite understand it. I print it out, sit for a while and go to bed. It is a tiny detached one-bed house, a former stable block with floor-length windows. It is very close by, opposite the park. From a 72dpi jpeg the doors look wide enough to take a wheelchair. It has a downstairs bathroom and seems to tick all the occupational therapist's boxes. I have walked past this house before and noted it with interest.

We could live there. Ev and I would sleep on the mezzanine and Tom's bed would be below in the light of the long windows. In the night we could talk to each other. Christmas is coming in a few weeks and this is fast becoming a problem. I think we should have a great Christmas and I don't think we can have it in hospital. So I am looking for somewhere to celebrate. Here is such a place. We could set ourselves up, invite everyone over and they would come. You could cook big meals and get in quite a crowd. It is expensive and risky I know. It constitutes a pretty mad plan but it is a plan. I am heartened to have two sheets of paper stapled together to wave at the meeting. I feel much better and I look no further.

The next day we assemble in the Relatives' Room that Ev has grown very fond of. The physios, the occupational therapist, a doctor I've not met before, the very young nurse, and an Australian social worker with a squashed face who I am told is assigned to us. I have not met him before either. Dr B's registrar doesn't arrive till ten minutes before the meeting ends and neither the discharge coordinator nor anyone from the palliative team is present but I don't realise this and it leaves the illusion that Aussie is the man responsible for getting Tom out of here. We have had no contact at all with the palliative team so I don't know if the lack of them is a problem or not. The meeting kicks off an hour late and though this is tough on a terminally ill patient having to sit around in a wheelchair, we are in a fine black humour so we do not mind. I show him my little stable and his eyes widen happily to circles in amazement. Tom's face is a mobile comedy. His eyes, assisted by his eyebrows, do a deal of work. They are like anemones reacting lightly to the environment: tiny changes in the sea's temperature, plankton shoals, warm currents or droplets of pollution coming their way. They can open to twice their size and wrinkle deep into his face in laughter. They can hold your gaze. He thinks the stable looks funny and great. Tom believes implicitly in my capacity to find a way forward. Because he believes it, I do too and this is fitting. We are together. We will see what these people have to say.

When the meeting starts, Aussie is bullish and he takes centre stage. Once we have established that our home is not adaptable, his next sally is to say we would not want to touch any of the nursing homes in the borough as they are pretty shit. He uses the word shit. Someone in the room remonstrates mildly with this attitude but only weakly. The dialogue so far seems to go like this. Tom can't stay in hospital. Tom can't go home. Nursing homes are unthinkable.

Later there will be a groundswell of opinion against Aussie and his negativity prompts an internal inquiry as to what kind of a piece of time-wasting this conference is. Later I will get to tear his head off on the phone and kick his abject apology to pieces but today he is not contradicted. It is clear that no one else has a plan. Because I do have a plan and because an impasse is no use to us I get out my estate agents' papers and wave them about. I say flatly that the only way I can get Tom out of here seems to be if I pay for it. There is silence. Tom laughs. Aussie says if we had a house that worked then

Tom would be looked after by an increased community care package. Another silence. I laugh. I run quickly through the inadequacies of the community care package we had before entering hospital. Aussie says they are the better of the two on offer in the borough.

The meeting is inert. A sticker on the window says *Dust Sealed – Do Not Open*. People who work in institutions may recognise this as commonplace but I have never worked in such an institution and I do not. I don't understand what is going on. Including the time it took for everyone to muster, this meeting takes up an hour and forty minutes of seven very busy people's time. The professionals in the room defer collectively to each other. Aussie fills the breach. Two of them do not speak at all, including the duty ward doctor, who positions her chair as a doorstop, with one of her legs outside the room, clearly willing the rest of her body to follow. Dimly I understand that lack of leadership and the absence of the registrar or anyone with the authority of Dr B is a problem. Only a while later do I wonder if it is we who are the other problem. We appear to be enjoying ourselves. We might even be said to be relaxed. We present such a united front as to be impenetrable. Perhaps we are taking it too lightly. Perhaps we look like we can handle whatever happens to us, so our problem never seems acute. This is difficult. For us, remaining ourselves for as long as possible under these conditions is an intensive form of play, an art. This is what we do. I know this is what Tom is doing. He puts energy into it but it is not really a stretch. I match him. Together we are a combined puzzle.

Some simple formulations are missed out at this conference that would have served me well. The phrase, *Tom requires twenty-four-hour care*. This is a clear enough concept to put into a sentence based on the visual evidence but in the conference nobody says it and I do not hear it spoken until a week later when Karen, one of nurses, uses it as a retrospective statement of fact and I blush red to hear it so casually articulated. *Of course he does, what a fool I am.* Another phrase that is not used is: *The community care package does not apply overnight*. This is an equally simple proposition, known to most of the people in the room but not to me. It is not spoken either, so I go away with my Christmas stable and get ready to build it on paper, to make it work.

3.4

Ev is on the fulcrum of madness. Having just woken up from an afternoon sleep, he is seesawing about.

Want chicken, don't want chicken, not like that, not a bone, want a bone, Noooo, nooooo, want chicken, I'm tired. NO.

Calm down, calm down.

I can't calm down I'm afraid.

We are all upset, it's very difficult, Ev, and you are doing so well, so well. I know you are upset about Dad.

No I'm not. I'm upset about chicken.

Conversations with Ev are mined with devices. Invisible until you are upon them, they can blow up either way, thrilling like an unexpected flare, a burst of surreal confetti or so painful they punch my brain into paleness. Now he is dancing in front of me in the hall, waddling about with a full nappy swinging from side to side. *When I do this, my poo rolls about in my nappy having fun*. Poo is power with

Ev. He will not allow it to fall out of his body into a void and insists on using a nappy to keep it close and safe long after he has mastered using the toilet to wee in. I am stressed and bored by this. This habit can be true with boys in general. I have no way of telling if it is more particular to Ev.

To look at him it is not evident what our daily traumas are doing to his psyche. Nothing is hidden from him. Everything is played out in his sight. But this means that he is a watched child. I am vigilant for warning signs, physical changes or minute recalibrations of behaviour that might indicate anxiety. But on the surface of his long, clean body there are none. He does not develop eczema or withdraw from play. He does not become aggressive to other children. He does not stop eating. But all is being evaluated in his mind and the thing Ev could do as soon as he could talk about anything was talk about us. Withholding his own shit may be his defence. Articulacy is his line of attack.

Ev, let us try and sit on the toilet to do a poo.

No.

Tell you what, just come and sit for me for two minutes, you don't have to do anything, just to remember what it is like.

NO.

Why not, Ev, what's the matter?

I am worried about Dad's tumour.

I can tell from the view of his face askance to mine and the tone of his voice that this is Ev playing his master card. He is trying something out and doing it supremely well. He knows it will work. It is a wild card. The linkage between these things at any moment may be less secure than he claims. But it is unanswerable. Ev, you play like a genius. To say *I am worried about Dad's tumour* is to win any dispute he is involved in. I will always, always, back down. Any adult would. He's a real pro. *We are all worried about Dad's tumour, lovey, but poo is poo and tumour is tumour.* This results in a little breakthrough and he does come and sit and we chat about nursery; about what we had for lunch; HMS *Belfast,* where we go as it's next to the hospital and the small, leaf-choked runnel we played in today. After a couple of minutes he gets off, saying. *It's not working. I'm not a grown-up.* This is much nearer the mark. To resist the movement out of babydom with all its impetus away from me, away from skin and softness leaning against each other, towards having to do the dull thing for yourself in a little room in private. This is all understandable.

I have been left with this child, a changeling before time. He was never meant to be mine alone. Ev is a confluence child: a child of two tribes. He has that air. This morning very early I cut his hair, transforming him from imp to page. He is easy to please: I bribed him to sit still with a box of raisins. Quite often we spend the evenings alone, just the two of us. Exhaustion is a big factor. Partly I like it that way, partly I can't be bothered to ask for help and partly the help you don't ask for has waned. I am trying to think about how we are going to be but our mode is a threesome and this dictates the whole of its dynamic including my thinking on it. It is like the mainland trying to imagine being an island.

The child will remain by my side when the trio we are has gone. It is a small, good sign that I can still care for him and by this, in covert ways, look after myself. Tonight I eat spoonfuls of pesto from the jar out of the fridge and finish the leftovers on his plate. He sits on the sofa ready for ice cream after another long afternoon in the hospital. It is eight o'clock but our schedule is wayward and supper has been eaten on my knee by the fire. *Would you like some ice cream? Yes. Did you buy it?* He asks. *Yes*. He gives me an unaccountable grin and a shiver of delight shims along his naked legs into his toes, setting them kicking. I laugh into the freezer. He is lucky that boy. God he has luck.

Wherever we go, Ev and I, though we do not go far, our faces are turned to the ward in the sky like a signal tower. It calls to us every waking moment and asleep I would know its orientation. It is our magnetic pole. Ev is conscious of this in his own way; curious, fractious, accommodating, amiable, anxious, and I understand it in a kind of mechanical, task-based totality. I am with Tom when I am not with Tom: driving, thinking, fetching, carrying, listing, remembering.

Tom's position is so fixed in the bed that he cannot see the view extending out over the south but he catches the sun balls that go down these days in flames over the other, metropolitan side of the building. From the eighth floor you see the clarity of St Paul's unimpeded as Wren would have it, the dark tower of Tate Modern, the river, the wheel. Snow is on the way they say. The days are getting colder. The days are great and terrible. Great because he can still phone me and laugh and talk at me in his thick, rich voice. Like I said, no edges. He is blurring, borderless, bespoke: nearing a liquid state and his voice is a deluxe manifestation of this. Terrible, because now he is in the hands of others forever and separation from home is official. There can be no other way. Yet separated, in tiny slices, I can begin, ever so slightly, to be with him again. I am free from the burden of stopping him falling, or slurring, or fitting, or fretting, and I can sometimes, not often, for there are always legions of things to be done that cannot wait, but sometimes, come and be close. On the bed we sit attached by headphones, one ear apiece and listening. Ligeti ascending: a telephonic call sign to the stars.

The pull of the bed is elemental. We don't want to leave it but people say we must, so for one night it is arranged. On the Saturday morning as we are leaving, I stop by very early to drop off some clean clothes. Weekends on the ward are slow. When I get there the curtains around his bed are closed but I am rushed so ask to go straight in. *Of course*. Flicking back the curtain I squeeze myself into the space at the foot of the bed.

Tom sits upright, cropped and foreshortened, propped on pillows. Three women from three different continents are giving him a bed bath. The water is blood-warm with drops of oil. Wet cloths and dry towels. One moisturises his legs in long, lazy motion. Another cleans his nails. Four heads are bent in conversation. In the busiest hospital, in one of the densest cities in the world, they have all the time in the world for each other. At seeing me, his face lights in greeting. *Aaaaaah! Hellllooooo!* Their voices rise to meet me in warmth and pitch. *You don't need to hurry,* they say. *You can stay*. I do not wish to leave. I do not ever wish to leave. I do not want it to end. He is at the centre of attention, relaxed, simply enjoying himself. Everything is all right and will be now and forever. Ev is waiting for me below. I must descend.

I embrace him and as I slip away the curtain falls behind me sealing them in. In my mind they are there still.

Our destination is a friend's house in a trough of land with no mobile signal. The sky is overcast, solid, dirty weather, rain like spit. It is very cold. Nightfall sets a curfew on the village and very little moves save at the entrance to the pub. Each house has a vast and splendid television.

There are certain times when I most like to speak to him: mid-morning, around teatime, and again before lights out on the ward. The code is that when he wants to speak to me at any time he sends a blank text and I call back immediately. We call each other all the time. My friends direct me to a low bank of earth just off the road at the entrance to the village. If I stand on the topmost mud, with luck I will get a signal.

It is dark save for the moon, my companion, the one that has dogged me since all this began. The signal comes like a fragile miracle. One mark flickers on the phone, then two and then the man's voice is like another. I wrap myself in my coat and his funny, viscous words glug into my ear slow as a drunk. He is so happy to hear me. We are both undone. He uses his vocabulary – how many words does he have now, less than thirty? – like a grandmaster. I tell him about where I am on the mound, about the moon, the mud, and remind him of another time, long ago, in Scotland, when he did exactly the same for me: found a point of high ground each night so that his voice could reach me. It felt primitive then, from a folk tale about lovers. I send my voice freely into the dark for there is no one else to hear me. We say goodnight and goodnight and goodnight and use up all the words we know for goodbye.

3.5

The tumour's physical presence has grown. The little lump was only the start. This is unusual. Most people are dead before the thing shows itself. Disease has taken the weakest route via the scar to exit the head and is now flourishing outside the skull. This growth may be good. Better to be under our eyes where it can be dressed and assessed than couching inside, impacting on the skull, blotting out the brain. So, on the left side of his head above the ear is now something the size of a tennis ball. Or is it an orange? A potato? A chunk of Play-Doh?

The very earliest ad-hoc descriptions of the nascent tumour on screen were made variously by scanners, doctors and neuros, all choosing words to convey its interior presence on a subjective scale. Pea, they said then. Grape. Marble. Bead. They might have said pearl or baked bean or Malteser. Lychee. In the last weeks – or is it days? – the lump is much bigger than all of these things and it looks angry. It has a mean snakehead, red and yellow. It is about to break the skin. Then we will have more troubles.

This is what cancer looks like. I did not know that it could grow outdoors with cells burgeoning in the air like a plant, but then I was ignorant of all of this. Once I saw a great weed, a buddleia, growing out of a window frame on a Glasgow tenement, wild and unchecked, huge against the sky. It seems accurate to say it looks just like human matter: thick, dark, bloody, lumpen. This is what we are made of.

And if I said to you now that we three are together and we are happy. If I said that in a way we do not care at all about this lump thing because what has happened to us has already happened long ago and so much of the rest that has happened since then has been stuff made and lived through by us entirely. Would you believe me? So it is. This is, I repeat just so you remember, the good bit.

3.6

I have had a brain episode. Odd. The fast-flow lava of stress, red and black, has cooled to a crust over the molten stuff beneath and the friction between the layers causes something to happen. There is a limit to my mind. You should know that my task this month is twofold. I need to find somewhere for my husband to die and I need to find a primary school for my child. The deadline for both is now. For reasons I can't add up, a collective flip, category confusion, renouncing of responsibility, ineptitude, temporary system failure or a rotten social worker, I do not have adequate or in fact any help to find the first of these things. The second one alone is difficult enough in London so I have heard.

I am not on any mood-stabilising drugs. Maybe I should be. The episode occurs after a late-night call with Dr B. The call itself was not a shock, nothing surprising. It only solidified my understanding of care in the community as mirage. But the conversation has a backlash. I do not get away unscathed. I go to bed straight after and as my head goes down, the room swirls, circling and giddy in the dark like a nasty bit of drunkenness. This lasts a couple of minutes. After a while I fall asleep.

The next morning my skin has become autonomous. It is *live*. I feel its peculiar defection as soon as I am conscious. I am wearing someone else's skin. It is not dormant but ON, sparking with tiny electric impulses. Pricks and shocks are going off, on the soles of my feet, in my chin, the right side of my shoulder and down the back. This fails to ease or go away through the day. Clear thought is beyond me. I am unable to concentrate at all. When I try to engage with Ev I am conscious only of the nerves exploding along my arm. Sharp stabs attack the soles of my feet when I walk. This is so unnerving I cry out aloud. It can happen anywhere, at any time, so I must be alert and on watch, but for what? I cannot stop it. Like an idiot game against myself, the flesh is mobilised. The Numskulls are dropping acid. The body has sent out teams of Lilliputian bowmen and they are reconnoitring inside me. What switch can we hit next? *Fire!* Where can we attack? *Here!* Whole communication systems are going mad along my arm and down my back. I have injected live electric glitter.

I try to calm it, talk myself round. *OK, this is your body saying it has had enough. You could think of it as an extension of consciousness, a sort of commentary on being alive. The body says, 'Look – here is your foot. This one – see here, Fire! This is your shoulder blade.' It's just a heightened form of awareness. You are being reminded of these body-parts. It's insane, yes, but you might learn to live with it. You live with worse already.*

My motivational speech tails off. I haven't wit enough to keep it going and the electric critters keep rioting. I am depressed. I am going to die. I have MS. I have some hideous neuropathy. It could happen, you know. It would be just bad luck that not one of us but two goes. It's not impossible. My sole ambition is to live and the bar is low. I want to survive till Ev is twenty. That is my goal. Just so he is not too sad. So I can stroke his head some more and hear him tell me about his day. Don't mind really about anything else.

I get myself to the GP – good Dr F – and he organises a clutch of blood tests: calcium, cholesterol, liver, kidney, iron, some others I forget. Eight labelled tubes of dark blood go out and eight results come back some days later totally normal. *Stress*, says Dr F. *Stress*. You need two squares a day and time for yourself or you will go down the plughole or words to that effect. I say, *I know.*

It is so very easy at this point not to eat. My mother sends a food parcel. Vivien knows that if she places a piece of food in my hand, a sandwich, a pie or a vegetable tart, I will eat it and she acts accordingly. Otherwise I will not. I feed Ev. I buy food and make sure he eats but for myself, I don't mind, or more strongly, I don't care. I am not hungry.

Facilitator, gateway, guardian, custodian: I am the one people turn to for all the practical issues to do with Tom. *Where has the wheelchair got to? How does he like his coffee? Have you got any clean shirts? Would he like a visit this afternoon?* Or, speaking to him, *Do you want an orange juice? Yes. Can you not work the DVD player? No. Did something annoying happen on the ward? Yes. Shall I bring in some supper? Yes.* I am completely snared by the quotidian and its ceaseless requests. Thinking and feeling are exorbitant demands, well over the odds. There is little uninterrupted space with Tom. Not from visitors – let them all come – but it is simply so much quicker for him to get me to understand what he needs and sort it than to start laying out his basic blocks of language for someone else.

I resent this. There has to be more. But the big concept – our future separation and how we might express our feelings about it to each other – is beyond my thinking. We try. *You must understand. I too am not fluent. I am speechless.* There is no time. This is true and damning and in one way it might be a blessing but doesn't feel like one. My thoughts run on managerial lines. Management. God. Insane. Let all of it go to hell. Let it all go to hell and me too for the space of just one conversation about love and death and disappearance.

And yet ... Yesterday, home after an atrocious day, I get a phone call, late and long as ever from him, hailing me in a strong and boomy voice. *Do you feel well?* I say. *Yes! YES! You sound fantastic, my sweetheart. YES!* I am ecstatic. He can hardly speak for laughing. I ask him about what he feels, about the extraordinary sensuous curtailment and corruption of his body. We are both roaring as we speak, me on the sofa, him on the eighth floor, phones jammed hard to our ears. I go to bed wrapped in pleasure. He has had the paella I left in a thermos. He has eaten well. He has had his visitors, the evening's random good companions. He has communicated with all. His spirits are high as ever and my equilibrium, after a murderous start, is climbing fast to meet him, just as my day is rolling over and I lose consciousness.

3·7

17 November 2010

Dear Friends

This is a call among you for advice. Tom is still in Guy's. His spirits are very good. He is thinking, talking, his language very tricky but seeming stable. He wants above all to work on writing projects, and with friends to help, he can. We went out to the Courtauld last week to see Cézanne's Card Players.

But he is not at all mobile, he is in a wheelchair, and he needs 24 hour, quality nursing care. Which he is getting.

Tom is still very much himself. His coherence, and state of mind defy the visual evidence in his brain.

We are now looking for a nursing home where he can be comfortable and cared for, that will allow him privacy, safety and access to friends and preferably be not too far from Ev and me. I am out of my league.

If any of you have positive experiences of nursing homes in London, or any suggestions at all to make, please do pass them on.

Tom looks forward very much to seeing you. Those of you who have seen him lately know that he is a pleasure to spend time with. He loves your visits. One-to-one can be better for him than groups.

I send you all, our love.

If this were fiction, by this point it would resemble a badly plotted folk tale somewhere midway. It is gargantuan and over-complex. Its internal logic collapses under too many layers and it teems with characters, false trails and sisyphean tasks. I am in a car going around London with Vivien to look at nursing homes so that Tom can be discharged to a place where he may die. I am being pushed towards this option though that's not quite right, as option suggests choice and this is the one idea but nobody is pretending to be enthusiastic and I catch the tone correctly. Somewhere about the hospital is a Mr Discharge who gets mentioned a lot. Everyone says I should meet him as he's the key man but no one arranges it so I don't and time goes by. We are finally connected to the hospital palliative team and I am regretting it. Palliative comes to see us every now and again. Yesterday she mentioned in passing at our bedside that there was a good nursing home for younger patients in Tunbridge Wells but when I closed my eyes to slits and turned my reptile head towards her, letting my gaze brush her ever so lightly, she paled and weakened and withdrew to another part of the ward.

My flesh is morbid. The epidermis jangles with static in a continual electric burn, a low fire on the tundra of my arms and shoulders that sometimes licks into the air on the scalp under the hair. I have no faith in this project. Muscles, eyes and tongue tell me. I am not mad. I am sane. I taste the idea of separation and the weakening of our orbit around each other and the taste is bitter. My body is in permanent revolt. I do not eat, my shit is black, but here we go in the car to check things out, as really, what do I know? I am a Lay Person.

And should this nursing home be what we are to do, should our options be so curtailed, well then, we will track down the one place in the whole of the city to suit us. A folk tale like I told you: a fairy story. This is probably the only day on which I know that I am in no condition to drive. I do not say this to Vivien.

We are at the limit of knowing what to do. A terrain where my guess seems as good as theirs is at such high altitude that I am deprived of oxygen. There is no system here. Following the case conference a young ward doctor sweetly gives me the name of a nursing home. He gets the address off the Internet and writes it down on a bit of paper in front of me. It's the one he knows (... *and the others, the ones more suitable for a young family, the ones suitable for someone with Tom's complex medical needs, or the ones not exclusively for geriatrics?* ... so many questions, but this time I am silent). We decide to target this one first off but see it together with another picked at random on the Internet for comparison. You'd do that if you were buying a fridge or a car or a new hi-fi. We are choosing a place to send my husband away from his family to die. I hold the piece of lined jotter paper in my hand like a black note in a story by M. R. James. So well meant, it is terrifying. In the car I look at it again. It says, *There is no system for you. You are falling as well as dying.*

Home One is nearby, a big plus. The ladies are warm and kind to two enquirers pitching up. They are proud of their place and want to sell it to us. I like them. I believe in them. I like the good feeling they give off: of love for their patients, friendliness, adaptability. They will make it work for us! Together we can do it! They dole out attention and humour. Guests trot by with little dogs to visit relatives.

The building is a single storey overshadowed by high flats and its corridors and corners get no light. It must have been built before the difference sunlight makes to the brain was fully recognised. The edges of everything are set too close to the edges of everything else. All verticals are bumped, bashed, scraped, eroded, as if minutely chewed away from the inside. The rooms are tiny, small as can be, but there is one, a strange sort of double, bigger than the others, that I am led to understand is available to those who can pay a supplement. I inhabit it in my imagination in an instant. I am expert at this kind of makeover. Yes, we could do this and this, bring a lamp in here, a bed for Ev, take that out, paint this, change the rug. They make encouraging noises. They are sympathetic, keen to help.

The building fronts on to a car park. Architects call it hard landscaping but those who are not architects have no name for it. It is set so low that the windows offer no solace: not a single tree, no promise of sky. I have a vision of carrying Ev screaming into the place by force. There are no doctors on the premises. This is of course standard with all nursing homes. *Why are we here again?* My lack of belief in what we are doing muffles my thinking. It disables me. Tom's body fails in all sorts of complex ways all the time, from the banal – immobility – to the extreme – the volcanic excrescence growing above his ear. These different ways of failing are not set to get better. Already he sits rapturously at the centre of a tight tornado of medical attention, soaking all of it up, day and night.

The second, Home Two, is fancier. It resembles a middle-market hotel you might end up in if you were passing through a town and didn't know anyone. I have stayed in such a place on the outskirts of Leeds. It has valances, complicated curtains and too much furniture in every room. Here the ladies don't seem to mind so much whether we come or not. The furnishings are in the international, institutional colour you see a lot of, a rusty-red yellowish brown. They call it sienna. Dried blood is what it is. Someone should tell them. This home is much bigger and the staff more impersonal but it looks well run and trim with a tight and shapely designer garden they are very proud of. There is more light and personality to the spaces but the baseline noise throughout is channel-war. The everlasting death-battle of daytime television plays out at a volume set for all to hear. It is violently hot. The residents, as in Home One, are uniformly very old. The same medical care conditions apply. No doctors.

What will happen to Tom when he has pain at the moment he has it in one of these rooms painted in shades of old blood? What happens when he can't move his arm to operate the call button and no one can hear him over the television? I cannot live with him here. Ev cannot live with him here. I have another vision, this time of me, being led weeping, inconsolable, out of the place.

To them we must appear like regular folk making a decision. To see us, you would think that we were weighing things up, having a choice. Far away from all this but nearer to me than any of it is Tom, my near-wordless, supremely articulate companion, my brain-damaged, highly intelligent dear-love, still so at home in his personhood and his drifting body. My husband who knows that he is dying, his intelligence fully stimulated, awake and improvising all the while fresh and exotic ways of being in the world with us. I am stunned. We get into the car and drive.

I am slow, but I start to understand the day's work as a piece of administrative filler. It is a formality. No hospital stay can be open-ended. The EDD, the Estimated Discharge Date box on the whiteboard, though it may be wiped and re-scrawled many times over, needs a date at any given moment or questions will be asked. A plan is forming. It is to do nothing. None of this will happen. I won't let it. It is wholly inappropriate for us. Why they won't acknowledge this to me is a puzzle but not my problem, though I can see that I am theirs. We are in a position of strength. We cannot be moved from our square metres of ward by force.

So far I have told Tom everything that happens. But I never recount this day to him. It is a secret I do not break. I do not speak to him about Home One and Home Two and I hold my fire about the other place, for slipped between these two experiences was another: a digression on the road.

On the drive from One to Two I saw a street sign, so small I hadn't noticed it before. *Hospice*: pointing left. My path went to the right. I should have gone to the right. Without thinking I signalled left. Friends had told me about this place. *Let's take a look.* I slid the car round and into a waiting bay. There was a gravel path and a door open to a reception area in a blue-grey colour with tall windows behind backing on to a lawn. We did not go further than the reception. No one stopped us but we halted and stood there for a bit, looking about. I noticed my breathing: acclimatising, checking in. We did not speak.

The receptionist was on the telephone. On the desk was a spray of sharp Christmas grasses edged with white. She finished her call.

Can I help you?

How can we come here? I asked her.

…

I am looking for somewhere where my husband can die.

I leaned in, elbows on her desk, eager to edit the story down to bullet points so she might process it but trying not to overwhelm her. It didn't work. Halfway through, a man in a white coat appeared and she hailed him and segued off in the same motion, leaving us together. So I began again with him, this time more slowly. I gathered Vivien to me. The three of us did not leave the desk.

I never learned this doctor's name. But when I spoke he nodded. I told him about our task that day and how I despaired of it. I told him about the note on torn paper. When he spoke we nodded. He told us that we couldn't just walk in: he spoke about referrals, procedures and time-scales, about Primary Care Trusts and funding. He asked about our trajectory, where we were, who was looking after us and what had happened so far. *Yes. Yes.* I said. *OK. I see. And how does that work? Yes. OK. I understand. Right. Yes.*

The conversation took ten minutes. *Thank you*. The three of us shook hands. We did not ask to look round. We got into the car.

Back at the hospital I put my plan in place. I say nothing and I am not asked. I take no more initiatives. I do not pester anyone for names of nursing homes or try to find any more houses. I do not ask for more advice and interestingly none is given. I just let it go. It is sweet. Ten days pass and I am passive on the subject of the future. We live, Tom in the hospital and me and Ev outside it with the daily runs between joining us all together. We are surrounded by a galaxy of nurses while the orbit of friends around us turns and turns. I am much happier.

After ten days we know that the tumour is advancing. Avastin is not working. Things are shifting, turning, widening. Each stage is marked and definable yet without a clear edge to guide us. There is nothing at all to grab hold of.

It is mid-morning and I get a phone call from Dr B.

How are you getting on with nursing homes?

He is not going into a nursing home.

What do you want to do?

I want to go to the hospice, to Trinity.

Then that is what we will set in motion.

Can I tell him that is what we will do?

That is what we will do.

3.8

Pain. He is in pain. Sub-cut morphine. We are adrift, stranded on an ice floe until someone rescues us and brings us back. I cannot write on pain so pain does not get written down. It is blank. The nerveless nature of the brain means the interludes of pain have been mercifully short and recent but for their duration I have nothing to say. They lie in the white spaces on the page.

This is where Tom's lack of words bites hardest. When he can only indicate what is wrong and have us guess at its extent and urgency and guess what we can do to alleviate it. Pain takes up various positions and attitudes. There is the pain of not being in control of the body: to live as weight and mass and be moved not under your own volition. This is exhausting. There is local, temporal discomfort; maybe a limb is in the wrong position or a cannula has been pulled too tight and snags across the skin. When we discover this kind of cause we feel elated. So easily remedied! Only this! We almost dismiss it. But it is pain. There is hurt from the cancer visible since it has become a wound apparent in the flesh. There is mental distress; the thought that perhaps the pain might not go away, or not go away soon enough, then what next? Sitting upright for too long is agony. There is extreme fatigue from living in a mind stretched to the horizons of being. It is all pain. Pain throws many shapes.

We go down to the river in the wheelchair with Ev and a friend. Tom is in pain, but he had set the plan in motion well before the episode began and it's already taken two hours to organise to this point so he wants it to go ahead. I don't want to and we squabble. Rightly or wrongly I tend not to win. So we set out, two women, a young child and a man in a wheelchair. By the time we get to the river's edge every kerb and cobble is such an assault on the suspension of the chair and the integrity of the body that he wants to come back. So we come back. The damp air is treacherous on our faces like a wet towel pulled tight over our mouths. The city is pallid, fogged, shut down.

Tom has pneumonia again. This happens. To move is to operate the machine and to lie still courts infection and the capitulation of the lungs. He gathers his resources to fight and sinks into himself. High-end antibiotics against a menagerie of ills are prescribed. Physically he is very strong and I believe that only the tumour will beat him. Never for a moment do I think he will not win this one. I am not worried. This is a local fight. His drugs calibration has become acute. He is monitored hour by hour.

3.9

But Dad's not dead yet, he's still here.

We are sprung. Free. It is visionary as Blake: a sudden epiphany in the air above Lambeth. A bright motif, a shift, a star, a shape etched deep, historic emblem blazing within our narrow section of time. This is how it comes about.

In the hospital, for days nothing happens save the progress of disease and a barely controlled, gargantuan social life. Bureaucracy is at an impasse. Around Tom's care a constipated mass of people and agencies strain against each other, each trying to pass their own stool and execute their fragment of the whole but the whole then jamming under the impact of conflicting agendas to stall any decision. It is a confined space. Stasis. Pile-up. Uncertainty. Days pass.

In the confined space, vast now, is Tom. He casts a fierce light. For his friends he is a magnet for activity and action. Around his bed there is no more place to sit. He is not an easy person to place. I can see that. Today is a red flag day: signalled in advance. I go in very early as he is to be marked up by Dr B for radiotherapy in a final attack of electrons to the head. This is a holding measure, an attempt to stall the lump, and it will be the last intervention he will receive. We both understand this. I told him the news. No more Avastin. After more than two years of treatment there will be no more treatment. I say it again here. *No more treatment.*

The palliative nurse corners me just before we go off to be marked. Would I like to go into the Relatives' Room for a chat? I would not. What is it with Palliative? I have been around hospitals a while now. I am this building. My skin is rubbed transparent by it. My body is piping and ducting, my lungs the corridors through which I inhale its air. Its coffee is my coffee, its blood, my blood. My child has eaten food off its floor and still lives. I sense conflict. Someone's nose is out of joint. Palliative has learned of the hospice proposal from another quarter and there is something she thinks is not right. *No,* I say, *let's talk in the corridor*. I take up a position between the radiator and the fire hose, shoulder to the wall and feet planted against the contra-flow of staff nurses and sisters. If anyone tries to rush me here, I am secure.

Do you realise that people can only go into hospices for two to three weeks and after that, if they plateau, they will look for other places to move them to?

Then they will have to fight me.

What's wrong with nursing homes?

I do not have any confidence that they can care for the complexity of Tom's situation in a way that I want them to.

I think you should give the idea of nursing homes another chance.

The consultant thinks the hospice is now the right solution. She said that the window of opportunity for a nursing home has closed.

(I do not tell her I never believed it to be open.)

Consultants often don't know how the system works.

So you are directly contradicting her?

No, but I just want you to know the situation, people can't stay in hospices indefinitely.

This situation is far from indefinite. I wish it were. The consultant, who is the person I must trust in this, has the evidence of the scan. It is very bad.

You should also know that it might take weeks to get a place. Just as long as you are aware of this, you might be in this hospital for weeks.

Have you asked the hospice if there are beds?

No.

Then why don't we have this conversation in the light of fact.

I sound murderous but I am acting. Surprising. I feel slightly relaxed, detached. Something in the near distance is giving way, like snow dumping quietly off a pitched roof. I feel it. If I do very, very little, stick around, watch carefully, pay close attention and don't move until the time is right then we will win. The game is this. Either inertia wins or velocity wins. The stakes are at their highest. We need to get out of here while Tom still has the power to express his life. I am powerless yet I hold the cards. We will get what we want. We will win.

Tom's lump is marked up with pen and a black marker circle is drawn round it like an illustration in a Ladybird book. *Here is the lump. It is big. Look! Here!* I could have done that, or Ev. I am no longer interested in medicine. Medicine has done with us. I imagine it's like the arrows they draw on bodies before an operation to show which kidney to take out. But then the consultant and the radiologist start to exchange strings of numbers. They bring out stencils: circles, squares in different sizes to focus the rays and folds of lead to shield the ear. We are sidelined. I stroke Tom's hand as we chat. He is so tired but looks wild and brilliant. It's been a mad morning what with Palliative and all and we haven't even got to lunch.

As no porter is to be found, Dr B and I push the bed back its long return to the ward. Such a daft, comedy thing a bed, and so hopeless when pushed by amateurs. It goes nowhere we want it, into walls, steel doors, all edges converging, wheels in lock. Dr B is as bad as me. Tom is encouraging: alternately bored and laughing as he watches us smashing about. We tuck him into the sheets for safety. His limbs mustn't roll over the edge. While we are waiting for the lift I begin for speed to talk to Dr B out of his earshot when I notice his face go all funny and cross. He gesticulates and beckons us over. Stupid of me to make this mistake *now*. He is a person. He will not be talked over. We group around the bed and I repeat the fresh conversation with Palliative verbatim to Dr B. *That is not how it works*, she says. I nod. We will win.

Liberation, total and absolute! We are free. Very early the day after my encounter with Palliative she phones me at home. I have just dropped Ev at nursery and I am staring blindly out of the window, squinting at the shape of the day: same as all the days. *Tom has a place in the hospice, he will go today*, Palliative says. *Eh*? She repeats. I am silent. *He will leave at 1 p.m.* Suddenly I register what my eyes had been looking at before the telephone rang. Bright leaves of gold and lime are crowding and waving wildly at the window for my attention on the tree outside. I phone him immediately but he has already heard. Using a hand-made repertoire of torn-up words – *yes, no, on the other hand, indeed, also, then, God, want, I, but, maybe, good, well, oh* – he conveys fullest delight.

Do you know what this means? It means we have a future.

3.10

7 December 2010

Dear Friends

Tom moved today from Guy's, where he has been for five weeks, into Trinity Hospice on Clapham Common. We are delighted and relieved. It's an incredible environment to be in, to spend time in. We can be at home.

You are all welcome. There are no restrictions at all on visiting.

Nearest Tube, Clapham Common, is five minutes' walk.

We hope to see many of you on Thursday at Tom's exhibition at Victoria Miro.

With love

The hospital was vertical. Beneath us, stacked like ballast, was our fellow cargo: layers and layers of the metropolitan sick arranged in dense, industrious warrens of gut, heart, bowel, bone, blood. The hospice is horizontal. Its planes stretch out flat and space is not at a premium. Though not at ground level, it feels like it; you enter continuous with the land outside but at the rear, another floor is tucked beneath. Our room fits snugly into its level and looks on to the garden at the angle of a person looking down on his own shadow.

The building is new and fitted out in warm wood flanked by wall-to-ceiling windows. All is light from edge to edge. The large rooms come off a space that is not so much a corridor as a broad spine running the length of the building that operates as lounge, office, throughway, sightline and meeting place. The ideological imprint is one of openness. At no time do you have to knock on a door to search for a member of staff. Nothing is hidden.

Rooms can be porous or private as you wish. The interior wall is glass with blinds that open or close at the touch of a button and the exterior one is also glass and opens on to balconies. In summer the beds can be pushed outside. All areas save these rooms are held in common. Sitting in the public space I see the spout with boiling water on demand for tea. Cups are set out and waiting. There is a television with seating grouped around. Small bright green and blue chairs demarcate the toys area that is Ev's domain.

The building is temperate. To watch the nurses walk down its length in their short-sleeved tunics of white, dark blue or light is Mediterranean. It is a passeggiata so generous and deep that strollers can choose whether to acknowledge each other or not. No one is obliged. Sofas, seats, rugs, tables, flowers, giant photographs and bowls of sweets make stopping points along the way. Nurses eat sweets all day. The toys area and the most prominent lounge, signalled by two giant leather sofas in an L shape, are just opposite Tom's room.

They are technically in our lee and therefore ours, so often we take them over. Once again he has the lucky room, Room 1, at the head of the row next to the nurses' station. At night when he needs attention I stick my head out of the door and the nurses grouped there rise to cover the few metres between us. Their night-lit faces are serious to what I might say.

I feel like I have made contact with a closed sect whose mores I do not know. There is an openness and at the same time a discretion here that is hard to quantify. It takes me much, much longer to learn the names of the nurses. In the hospital there was Gail, Rebecca, Tayo, Nick, Sean, Rachel, Joanna, Karen, Angela. I learned their names in days. This was partly a group incantation, a recitation in praise and awe at their skill, but also to name is to know. I needed to note the ones I liked and mark how their identities were invested in their actions. What was the look on their faces as they appeared at the end of his bed? What words did they use to greet us? With what level of detail did they turn back his sheet? How did their hands work together to lift his right arm? I can count the number of bad nurses we have met on the fingers of one hand – would you say I was lucky? – the one from Streatham, the one who wanted to retire to Australia, the Dutch one, the angry one …

It was a promiscuous love. I would single out one as the most exquisite, easily the best nurse, and then another would come along more beautiful and I would fall harder in love again. My friends did it too. Each day the accolades flitted about. *She's the one – But no, what about her? Oh, I love her*. Finely blended with this praising was a more strategic aim. In the hospital we were in a vast system of competing needs where Tom had to be brought to their attention as a cause to be championed. Perhaps I didn't need to try so hard. He manages still, deep into his illness, to make friends and admirers directly. He attracts them. He is powerful enough not to need me. But my work was strategic: to be his proxy within the system, to find out who had power in it and who did not and most importantly who knew who had it. In Ev too, I held an ace in flagging up our cause. Ev carried them all before him. Nurses fell about in his wake.

Here I don't need strategy. Tactics are over. Power is level. I don't need to learn the names immediately so they take much longer to come: Holly, Mariana, Jasper, Emma, Charlotte, Amma, Rita, Cecily, Julie, Nigel, Delores, Barbara, Brenda. I don't need to make alliances to get what I want. What I want is visible. It is given to us. I can see it.

The nurses work on tables or at the long work station running down the side of the central space. There are so many of them it can seem social, as if they are lounging, doing light paperwork or puzzles, chatting, drinking tea, taking it easy. But they are working, and something about the way they hold themselves when they work tells you that you can interrupt them.

I don't have to make myself especially special. I don't need to get in early to catch a doctor on a ward round or risk missing a development for days. I live here. There is no crowd that Tom needs to stand out from. It will all work anyway. I can let down my guard. But this feels violently risky. It is not relaxing but disconcerting, like vertigo. I might fall over. We have been going at such a pace that to stop now feels too dangerous, too extreme. The last weeks have been so wild and hard-edged that in this place I am a barbarian: uncouth, uncivil, self-conscious of my raging desires. I want to drool and spoil and swear and make a mess. Tom is dying. This is a place where he can die well with us around him. Suddenly, overnight, we are home.

The room was already handsome before we began. But as you would in any new house, we make it ours. My first action is to bring in the standard lamp from home with the prefabricated shade I made by taping two shades together. This will be our beacon.

The long wall opposite the bed quickly becomes a solid screen of familiar signs: pictures, writing, drawings, photographs. This is my second action. I bring them in from home and he watches me work with pleasure and interest. He points things out as I stick them up or will ask me to move an image from one part of the wall to another in greater or lesser proximity to his line of vision. He is a curator. His aesthetic is in no way impaired.

I have a system for putting up photos. I don't know where it comes from but you can try it. It will adapt to any area. You start with an edge, here the one around the indent of the bathroom door directly opposite the bed, and you work with the whole wall. You line the edge with images, each butting up to each, no gaps. Then you work outwards and upwards quickly, like a professional, not paying much attention to what goes next to what, no attention to content, though some to abstract attributes like shape or density of tone. Key to the process is Leave No Space. Images of different sizes are fitted alongside each other so that their edges are roughly aligned for the next layer.

Collisions are fine. It is a dry-stone wall technique. The borders of the mass as it grows over the wall are indeterminate. They stop only when they hit an obstacle or when the whole goes out of the reach of my hand. I think about bringing in a ladder so that the pictures can go all the way to the ceiling but I don't get round to it, so I go as high as I can reach by adjusting the adaptable stool to full height and putting one foot on the sink.

So this is what he sees: a painting by Ev on sugar paper of a green horseshoe shape next to a red indeterminate figure with blue scratches. Heraldic. The poster from the Wyndham Lewis show we went to earlier this year in Madrid. Us on the evening of our wedding standing in the tunnel we made out of white tarp. A postcard of Blake's, *Help! Help!* from *For the Sexes: The Gates of Paradise.* Ev in France a year ago with the texture of the sun imprinted on his upturned skin. A photo of my old flat in summer when the plants grew so thick up the wall that from this angle the door is invisible. In the first four years of marriage we lived in both our flats. A recent picture of us trying to decipher something in one of Tom's notebooks. He is wearing his beret and the apron he wore to eat, the costume of his last month at home. Tom's print *Political*, made for his exhibition that will open tonight. Ev and I on my birthday two years ago. It was our first post-diagnosis celebration and my eyes are glassy. Thomas Bewick's engraving *Tail-piece for the Long-Legged Plover*. A still from *epic*, the film I made in Rome, the one with the horse. Ian Hamilton Finlay's *The Little Seamstress*. A rough draft for a card we adapted from Leger's *Holly Leaf on Red Ground* with the red ground removed. A poster of Poussin's *Landscape with the Ashes of Phocion*. A love heart card drawn by the twins. A print of the cover of the *Observer* Review that came out a month ago. It shows Tom and Ev sitting side by side like beanbags thrown on to the ground on the afternoon after Tom's first fit. Tom and me ten years ago, playing table tennis on my piece *Fresh Air: Hyde Park*. The piece is a one of a trio of table tennis tables in the shape of London parks. A line drawing of us mooching around Liverpool the year I was at Tate. Cézanne's *The Card Players*, a memento from the Courtauld trip. Ev with a bruise on his forehead looking like a righteous evangelist after a beating. Kitagawa Utamaro's *Lovers in the Upstairs Room of a Teahouse. A* 'child's' collage of Tom with a fur beard, done by me while bored at playgroup. A card from Blaze in careful felt tip. A postcard of the Uffington white horse.

Soon there are no surfaces left on which to put anything down. Piles of CDs, letters, books, medical stuff, flowers, bottles of wine, chocolate, accumulate on every surface. Our possessions bank up on the floor. Everything we are not immediately using I heap in the bathroom. The cleaners do their best and pick their way gently around us. Within days it gets out of hand. This is endemic. The nature of the situation is untenable, spatially, temporally and metaphorically, and in response the only thing we can think to do is continue to bring it in and continue to pile it on. As we go deeper there is always more to be learned. And we learn it better too. More and more time, more and more friends, more and more things, more looking, more speaking, more stroking, more sitting, more eating and drinking, although that is signalling itself to be the most untenable action of all. Tom's swallow reflex and the brain's ability to work the throat are breaking down.

The impact of our new home is so sudden it is impossible to make sense of. To avoid an accident, you brake, you do not crash, but find yourself thrown off the road into a place where you do not even need a car. This is how it feels. But the change will have a longer impact, like a slow fuse that may never stop. I am a pragmatist. I learn and I learn. We have many things still to do and we can do them here. Tonight is the opening of the exhibition of Tom's collage works at Victoria Miro. The works are highly crafted combinations of text and image made entirely of paper and created manually with scissors, a wax roller and a store of magazines. He was always a writer who made images. For five or more years these pictures were published weekly on the editorial page of the *Independent:* topical, arcane, satirical, political, celebratory, their scissored edges softened by reproduction but not their import. The originals have never been shown. It will be a great show. Twenty-five works framed around the high space. The invites have gone out. The press has been notified. It will be a great party. Tom is going. Holly the nurse is going. Ev is going. I am going. Everyone is going.

3.11

Who is this person? The same who loves me. The same I have lived around for fourteen years. Yet even so. He is asleep. Removed to a degree, too weak to impose himself much on his illness. Not too weak to breathe, no. The breath goes on strong though his chest is shallow rising and his cough full of fluid. A nurse described the lungs for me as an upside down tree with the trachea the trunk that branches further out and down into finer, separating, diffusing roots. Although his illness and he are one and always have been the same, prime space in the brain is being lost apace to the interloper. What size is the thing now, a clenched fist? Last night I slept at home and called him early. *Hello! Yes! Good!* … All very cheerful, his voice upturned and sane when I told him that Ev and I were on our way with bacon sandwiches and coffee. We are two days after the exhibition and we still glow in its after-burn but I sense that something is wayward with his eyes, a strangeness, a blurring, failing.

Around midnight I sit nearby in his wheelchair – *Dad's wheelbarrow,* Ev calls it. The room is alive with tiny interruptions: minute clicks and shifts syncopate the whirring hum of the air mattress inflating as it adjusts his weight in the bed. Night-lights beep, electricity is everywhere cradling the three of us in the palm of its hand: safe, warm, happy modernity. The profile of the bed is spectacular. It is a constructivist dream-divan, bed as high-end machine, beautifully turned and finished and capable of multiple positions. His sheets are white, stiff, crisp and never dirty. Swiftness of intercession here is all.

Tom's left hand clutches a beaker of water. The left has a strong grip still, though the wrist is bruised blue from months of bloodletting. The right hand is dormant. He looks like himself. He always looks like himself and as usual that means he looks well. Tonight we have been talking about the things people talk about when they do not have long to live. What will their children know of them? You might think this comes up all the time but no, it doesn't. There are so many other yet more serious and yet more frivolous things to crowd it off the agenda.

The conversation goes via our usual channels, starting with the elimination of every possible other subject – local, practical, conceptual, spatial, emotional. *Is it to do with food? Is it to do with how you felt at the exhibition? Is it to do with someone you met? Did it happen recently? Is it in the room now? Is it to do with love? Is it to do with your work?* Context provides a ragged map but consider all the subjects there are in the world and think about how you access them. It is hard to analyse such a thing. Something might enter your thinking, triggered from where you are not sure and quick as a flash you are on a new thought runnel in complete darkness, one you weren't even conscious of a second ago, that runs away directly from the main stretch. The route back is instantly opaque. The path ahead becomes illuminated only when you step on it.

A conversation is not like a diagram. The thing we cannot do is engage readily with the idea of a subject, so arriving at understanding is improvised, imperfect or impossible. It can take many hours and there is a high risk of failure. One of us, me or he, might well stop before we get there, might throw in the towel, get too exasperated or tired or bored, and say – as I do often now – *let's come back to that one* – or – *let's try again when we are fresh*. I use that word a lot with Ev, *Fresh. Sleep, darling, sleep, and you will be fresh.*

The next night I am at home. Incredible! It's midnight and he is calling me. I remember the first phone call I had from him. It was on the communal phone in the hallway of my bedsit and as we spoke my bare feet on the tiled floor wicked up the cold. That was a frigid house, stalked by the neurosis of the landlady, and I got out as soon as I could.

The telephone is as radical an agent of transformation for us now as it was then. That ring had such urgency, belling the insertion of promise into the deeply unpromising.

Now my phone shows the familiar digits ending – 101. *Yes!* Directly on hearing I understand everything. He has company: his thick Father Christmas voice, a scrunching in the background, laughter, the wrong digits beeping the phone, scroffling of pills and sheets, clumsy rumples of warmth, something being dropped, more laughter. How acute is the ear at picking up mini-tones, complex chords, small ambiences and sub-sets of meaning. I may yet be happy forever and ever as long as we can simply talk on the phone. Fantasy I know. No matter.

Tom's desire for company is insatiable so Tim has gone into the hospice very late to sleep over. They are having a glass of wine. I taste it with them on my tongue as I hear it: the noise of a sour, dense, rich little grape popping sweetly amongst the other little noises. I know all the pictures he can see. I know the room is warm and full of his things. I know that the Christmas tree outside in the garden is flashing white lights on rotation as it will do all night. I know all this. Twinkle twinkle. All is well.

3.12

Dad was in Guy's and he grew bigger and bigger and then he went pop and moved into Trinity.

The manifesto is in the architecture. The volume of the building sets out the fibres of the relationships within it. How we negotiate our way around mimics how we are with each other. It is in the impress of the outside upon the interior and what that transition feels like as we pass. It is in how the light falls inside on a winter afternoon. It is implicit in how swiftly Ev and his friends settle to play when they visit. It feels profoundly strange at this stage in the long game to be pitched out of a place where these things were nowhere on the list of imperatives and into an arena where they are the fundaments of experience.

The hospice is above all a designed space, bright and confident about its ideology. Coherence is readable in every corner and detail and the work of the nurses runs seamlessly alongside. People and place have common cause. To arrive for the first time is to have expectations and to have them met. This was what happened to us. We came in off the street and stood in the foyer. We didn't go any further.

But Ev is agitated for the first time on arrival here. It is as if with this move he has finally lost patience with us. Enough of this life you've been leading me on. Whatever your reasons, it's not fair. Stop it! Time to finish, time for Dad to come home. Now he repeats this over and over. *But I won't have Dad at home if he is here* … I say *Dad can't come home, sweetheart* ... endless, endless, to boredom.

Ev goes to nursery on his usual days but he sleeps and eats mostly with us at the hospice. When he is here he says *I want to go home* and when he is at home he cries *I want to see Dad.* I am scissored. There is no solution. I say home is with us and I am here with Tom so mainly he is here. Overnight there is a heavy snowfall and in the morning the white roads are gently cut to ribbons by the tracks and curls of tyres. I have only one journey to do, between home and hospice. It takes ten minutes by car and I can do it without waking.

We are about to set off for the hospice. Ev is in the back strapped in his seat and he is sleepy. He suddenly starts and looks round. *He's not here. I thought that Dad was here. I thought he was with us. It was just a joke of mine.* I do not turn the engine on for a long while and we sit in silence until he becomes restless.

Sometimes the place seems ours. Our friends treat it as such. Like an out-of-the-way hotel in winter or a new private club they have access to. Dying has made a charismatic social space. *I didn't have anything on this evening so I thought I would come down the hospice and see who was around,* says Kathy. Ev's friends call by. He takes over the toys area with his gang or they build his wooden London set on the coffee table and invade it over and over with the probes from outer space while the adults conference on the low sofas or stare at the monochrome garden fattened with snow. At dusk the entire wall is dark glass. It is the shortest day.

There is a filmic quality to our life: dreamy, drowned and saved. Many hours can pass and by extension days. I live out in the open, more or less all the time, with strangers whom I trust entirely, or at any moment – equally filmic – with sudden assemblages of friends who arrive separately and together. If they didn't know each other before, these friends, they do now.

I don't know what director is making this piece. Someone says Bergman: European, shot flat without affect but deeply charged, with a fondness for long shots, no cuts, ensemble scenes, dark comedy and the action geared always to the man in the bed even though he is frequently off-camera. I hardly see the other patients. I cannot take my eyes off us. Death is selfish. I don't know the protocols and it takes a bit to learn. Do you chat? How to begin? *How long's yours got*? Actually it is simple. Compassion is configured over and over in mute smiles, glances, bends of the head, tentative exchanges of gifts, yoghurts, fruit, bread, a tea drunk together. Tom is young and Ev is young and I am young, so we are ever so slightly exotic animals.

The snow adds to my absorption. It smoothes and silences the world and removes it from me by degrees. We could be anywhere. It is difficult snow, no good at all for modelling. Ev and I go into the garden to make a Snowdad that Tom can see from his bed. The snow is too dry. It will not stick together. We cannot ball it up off the grass to give it any height or body. So the figure we make is only a heap, a low mound that we dress with a beard and eyebrows of copper beech and pebbles for eyes. When we finish I suddenly recognise him. It is the wide, dish face of the green man in his winter ermine at one with the falling snow, with his sides sloping and softening under snowflakes even as we work. The snow sits for a long time on the lawn and when it melts, our little heap lives for one more day.

The length of a day is no longer the measure it was. Days are no more use as yardsticks, nor hours, nor afternoons. It seems rare to have had such multiple experiences of time jammed so hard together. It creates its own kind of luck, a weird and elastic buoyancy beyond the usual rules, as if we have been outliving ourselves all the while. In the hospital we were pitching down a vertiginous chute at dangerous speed. Where were we heading? The aim in retrospect was simply not to die there. Before that, in those weeks of trying to keep together at home – weeks, or was it months, how long? – neither time nor momentum was measurable. There will be an equation for it but I do not know it. We worked three, four, five times as hard to stand still.

I am not frightened. The only time I am afraid is when I think back to the time before. I look at the other hypothesis – the what-might-have-been scene – now that it has been folded up and put away, and I see that it contains the groundwork for years of sifting through wreckage, a lifetime of damage. Sitting on the sofa looking into his room I feel none of these things so that view is unfathomable. But it was a flicker away, so slight, a hair's width, less, that I am afraid. We three have escaped. I have the deep shock of the survivor.

The days have no point of reference, no signs or markers. We have been in the hospice for two weeks and the big marker, the opening of the exhibition, is in the past. I know it is the week before Christmas – another kind of marker, though not of our making and therefore less relevant. Within this temporal field our families and our friends signpost the days themselves by coming and going. They coalesce in shifts and vivid groups: my parents, Tom's mother, his sisters, my brothers, my neighbours, our friends, people I've never met before. Some stay for half an hour, some for half a day. Some come every day. Though they themselves are subject to all the pressures of the season, to us they appear freeform and tied to nothing save us. They face only our way.

3.13

24 December 2010

Dear Friends

For those who are nearby, Tom, Marion and Ev will be at home at Trinity Hospice on Christmas Day and over the holidays. Please call by for a drink or a chat, a walk, or a play with Ev if you are around.

For those further away, we wish you a lovely Christmas.

To all of you, our thanks.

With love

I am busy. There are a few things best done at 3 or 4 a.m. The lights go out around 10 p.m. and all is quiet save for the intermittent call bells that send the nurses padding off down the hall. They never run. Each room has a bell. The sound is like an electronic violin playing two notes, one answered by the other at a different pitch. The noise is designed to be insinuating rather than immediate, not alarming, but impossible to ignore. It has the hallmark of intensive testing. When we arrived it took me a day or so to place even what the sound meant within the fabric of the building. I will know those two notes for the rest of my life. I can sing them. D and C sharp.

It is the night before Christmas. Everyone is packed away. Tom sleeps and my baby sleeps on a portable bed in the corner surrounded by decorations, cards, bells and a small illuminated tree. He lies under his duvet covered with stars. Beneath the bed his stocking waits for morning, its profile packed and bulging like a snake devouring a goat.

I have had a late surge of desire to commemorate my group of three with material objects. They must have presents! This is the consolation of the real. All desires are acted on instantly. There is no time. I am in the lounge stitching a blanket for Tom. He will love it.

I bought two plaid blankets and I am cutting the letters of our names out of the green one and stitching them on to the red one. Tom, Me & Ev. I do the cutting fair enough and the stitching rough for speed. I will have the rest of my life to do it properly. A catalogue on my knee supports the heavy cloth so that I don't stitch through on to my dress. I am too tired for mistakes now. It is a big task, mad for the late hour, but the spontaneity of it feels familiar and exciting, like how things used to be. But it means that I have not stopped since dawn. I am still trying to keep all the opposing forces in motion. I know I will be defeated but even at this late stage I try still harder. We are all at it.

The second gift is a present from Tom to Ev and I found it this morning. I knew I was looking for something, a gift to our child from his father in his last days but I didn't have an idea what such a thing might be. The symbolism of the gift defies all categories of object that might be found. When I saw it I didn't understand how good it was but as soon as it caught my eye, I trusted it and bought it straight away. Over the day I like it more and more.

It is a set of three small tables made in the 1960s that stack sweetly one into another like a little sculpture, a domestic Donald Judd. Three forms: big, middle and small, with a neat-fitting tongue and groove mechanism that slots them inside each other. They function together as one hermetic shape and separately as replicas of that shape. They are a family and they fit: each three planes of a rectangle with edges smoothed on top. All hail the unconscious mind. All hail the world to have such things in it. All hail chance to set them before me.

The tables will be Ev's. One day I will sand them. Remove the yellowed varnish. For now they can be tunnels, mountains, chairs, tables, cliffs and islands. For a short while he will be able to wriggle his body through them and soon, after all this is over, he will outgrow the smallest. Later he will not be able to fit himself through any of them and maybe for a while after that he will lose interest. Then sometime in the future his interest will return in full and he can claim them back from me. They are solid. They will last.

3.14

I have had forty-six Christmases. This one starts in a normal way. Ev is the first person I see as my eyes open. Tom is the second. Intimacy is not simple. It is made. The nurses do not disturb us unless they have to. They value our privacy more than we do and keep their interventions to a minimum. Early in a morning they check the drug levels in the syringe driver, change his position in the bed and bring his porridge. Then later they wash him, get him up and dressed. I mix Tom's drink, help him eat and get Ev's breakfast. The only thing I miss that I do not have at this point is a good coffee. I will have to wait until someone brings one in.

We have had three Christmases with Ev and I recall the texture of each, but without effort he creates new habits so I scarcely remember how it was before his arrival. Ev opens his stocking on Tom's bed and helps him unwrap the blanket. Tom can still use his left hand. They pull a cracker. Tom wears the crown. Ev heaps the blanket over Tom's head and pulls it off. Tom's eyes crease with laughter. His shoulders shake.

What I am seeing is an exquisite artefact held aloft. In many homes Christmas is a ritual pattern of small occurrences, yet to make this one happen – the child, the cracker, the paper crown – in the only place where it might have had a chance of happening, multiple agencies have played a role. Opaque and transparent, I cannot count them because I do not know them all to count: consultants, surgeons, nurses, therapists, doctors, relatives, friends, colleagues, strangers, donors, supporters, volunteers. Tom and Ev on the bed are a rare work of culture, dazzlingly constructed.

This year the hospice is the place to be. Tom sits in a wheelchair in the lounge and our friends arrive bearing gifts. The L-shaped sofas fill. Ev rips into present after present. These are his consolation prizes. There are too many of them. I hide them in the bathroom unopened.

Friends bring food too. But food is losing its function. Something is going wrong and the going wrong has folded in quickly. In order to be swallowed, food has to be pulped and eating even small quantities of solids can cause spectacular, all-hands-on-deck choking with nurses summoned. The bacon sandwich I brought in on Saturday is treacherous today. We cannot have such violence in front of Ev. But in fact we just cannot have it. It is too debilitating. So we adjust and we invent, we experiment further and further and shift the way we think of food, towards alchemical blends and suspensions of creamy fluids rich in goodness. Food becomes about colour, hue and dye. A palette of sharp vert of mint and soft pea, pumpkin with saffron strands, beetroot mash, flaming carrot shot with turmeric or stringent red tomato.

But I forget Christmas dinner. I fail to register its significance and Christmas dinner for Tom comes as small pats of slurry in monotone shades. When you destroy the structure and texture of meat, roast potatoes and glazed carrots this is what is left: three mounds merging on a plate like a bad chart, a pictorial rendition of malice. He is grieved and for the following hours is knocked out of sorts. Mine isn't anything either – I hardly taste what I eat – but there is little solidarity one can make apart from endless just-right silken soups, rice pudding, or the panettone I mash in solace with alcohol and cream, poison for a diabetic but we are beyond that now. Drink is thickened and food thinned, all substances converging towards an optimum consistency, a nutritional medium medium.

We are shadow chasing. Food is losing its charge. All is separating out and the laws that govern us no longer govern him. Today he gives up the nebuliser for his chest as too intrusive. Let it all lie.

3.15

27 December 2010

The 28th December – tomorrow – is Tom's birthday.

He will be 53.

Do join us for a drink in the evening at Trinity.

x

One. One. One one. The first day of two thousand and eleven is spent underwater. All of us are drowned and those who enter the room to sit awhile become complicit in the drowning party. Tom's mother is here and his sisters. His chest sounds like a stream, not free-flowing but blocked, choked upstream by leaves, sticks and silt, like a hidden rill shrouded with trees and wayward hedges running down the side of a path in Hampshire. He showed me once this place: the ditch where he used to play. I sit by the side of him to watch and listen. Sometimes I hear the noise in another way. Then it doesn't sound like a stream at all but like a fire when wind blows fitfully over the embers in a fickle stoking of energy.

Where is Ev? I don't know. Somewhere. At some point, maybe it wasn't today but another day, Tom wakes and we look at each other. *Aaah. Yes.* I see you now. This looking is just as it was. I know it well. I feel its charge like a little current unbroken. Maybe I can feast off this in the time to come. Maybe it will last me till the spring or longer but I cannot rely on it. My memory is wasted, over-stacked with stuff, and my hoarding is erratic at best. My memory may fail me. Perhaps it won't be a sporadic loss but a totality. Perhaps I will forget everything that has happened in the great wash of the hereafter. The present will be overtaken soon enough.

Epic sleeping is new. They said it would happen and everything else they said would happen has happened so I believe this too and I understand what it means. The lack of appetite is shocking. His appetites of late have been drug-fuelled, byzantine, outrageous but no, eating shuts down quietly and quickly in a day, two, without a fight. He has nearly stopped drinking. I keep temptations to hand: puddings, soups, biscuits melted in milk, cakes soused in alcohol, but none can rouse him.

Yesterday, on the last day of the old year, we were busy. We took Tom out on the common in his chair. Ev ran ahead. The air attacked our lungs and the cold rushing to our heads after the warmth inside loosened us and sent us mad. Stalling at kerbs we levered his weight up and down and about. We were erratic and tried to go too fast. Tom was jarred. The rest of the day was spent with friends in rolling sequence, eating and drinking and staying up late like everyone else. Yesterday though was a year away and today is payback for the brain. Tom folds in on himself like a three-dimensional structure made of tissue onto which has fallen a fatal drop of water.

A new year has begun. Perhaps the one cruelty of this story is that after this, when I look on to the garden, it will look the same. There will be no outward sign. At death the world does not alter: no shift of earth or change of colour, no noise, no shimmer of light, no falling or collapsing of physical objects. The tree standing there will still stand. *Stay, stay awhile longer.*

Heather brings a celeriac soup with chestnuts. It is riven with bacon and warm seams of root.

I wake from a dream. It is my only dream of the last two years and not so significant at first it seems but then I'm not so sure. In the dream I am looking for a studio but the work I plan to do in it is precisely and entirely the work of mourning. I am shown one like many I have seen, with white-painted floorboards, neon strip lights, slightly down at heel, just fine. But the studio is submerged under water: far, far down. Dark water, dense with creatures in shoals, swarms and pods, fills the windows and presses on to the skylight above. There are fish of great size and whiskery mammals like primitive beavers gone wild in the deep. There are dugong, ancient porpoise and illuminated colour-saturated krill, creatures with trumpets for mouths and kissing orgiastic lips. There are fat, fleshy, nameless things, fish with radiant internal architecture and skeletons of glass and giant anemones or maybe squid trailing filaments in foliate loops. They are ecstatic, pressing and magnifying themselves against the glass on all sides. They rub and fondle past each other and then retreat to become tiny opaque blobs against blackness, with new creatures ever coming forward to replace them. The water teems with their impossible numbers, all drawn out of the darkness by the single bulb of the studio light. *I like it.* I say. *I will take it.*

I had promised Tom a fish soup and as soon as the kitchen opens at midday I go to the French place with my flask in honour of the dream. We had eaten it there years before and I remember the viscosity as being just right for his throat. It is a real bouillabaisse, made of crushed warm little fishes, bodies and bones suspended in red oily stock, with no flour, no hidden thickener, the best for miles around. Talking to the chef I have the urge to tell him who the soup is for, as if to stress for him how much it means. But I don't say anything. It remains a transaction. Soup. In a flask. I do the errand and hurry back. He eats three teaspoons before he stops. I rub his neck at the place pressed and tucked against pillows where it angles into his back and get small sighs of delight. *Stay, stay awhile longer.*

Ev back from play brings in three sticks from the common. He lays them on the stool beside the bed. A present. Big, medium and small – he knows our configuration by heart.

This evening we have a little party. A small group come by for wine and songs. Tom knows the friends who come this evening. To each one's touch and greeting he utters a different sound but his eyes are closed. Only when he hears the voice of Ev at his homecoming does he open them. I see this. I am the only one who does. I am so very lucky. I might have turned my head to catch something and I would have missed it. I see that look. Their reach to each other is unchanged.

3.16

Thinking of a history of Death's depictions I can think of none that resemble what is happening here. Who is he? For a start a man: the ancient, skeletal, scythe-bearer, cloven-hoofed one, lord of darkness, thief, shadow. Our imaginings of him are puerile and simple-minded. They are pathetic, fantastical. They fail on every count. Where is the one-in-daylight, clearly seen; the functionary; the attentive one who commands all of our attention in real time; the one who withholds, withdraws; our symmetry; the one we call *Nature*? Childbirth is nothing. Death is mighty. The 0 to our 1. There is nothing in the world like it. But there is nothing in it that is not like the world.

I had thought that death was a separate, foreign state. It is, but it follows the contours of our own terrain. And because we knew this terrain so intimately we were able to continue on through it as allies. What we need to know here is what we already know.

On Tuesday, Tom goes to sleep. His breathing is natural and ordered. His face relaxed. I am here as ever and the others continue to arrive. Clichés of the bedside unfurl like mottoes out of our mouths. We are like medieval angels saying our allotted lines through the ages. We cannot help ourselves. *He is so calm. See how he sleeps.* If he could react truly he would roll his eyes, groan and tell us please to shut up. But it is true and mildly stupid at the same time. *Just wake up*. The colour in his cheeks is fresh. Daft. Like he could.

When watched closely like this, watched out as if your own life depended on it, death is normal. It is a series of stages more or less known. Here is a person asleep who will not wake. His breathing is not unstable. One. Two. One. Two. I pat the belly curve and trace the angle of its rising that I know so well, higher now than it has been but still. There there.

This quality of regard is not possible to maintain. It is beyond me to hold a coherent line or keep my thoughts in check. This becomes a prickly kind of ethical problem. It is a symptom of limbo. *Concentrate*. You may have no more time. *Concentrate*. But no, again, some nagging but persistent distraction has intruded: the new window I must order, someone who came recently, how hungry I am, thoughts of yesterday evening, my weeping right eye, where Ev is, the volume of the music playing ... Maybe it's not the right music, maybe I need to change it?

Music. Perhaps his accompaniment, his exit will be against this manual work. The dragging of hair bows across strings, friction against tightness, reeds vibrating, air blown through holes, through tubes. Valves shut off and opening again, lips relaxing and contracting, finely calibrated objects hit. Metal on metal; wood on metal; leather on wood; padding on metal; pitch, tone, timbre; cylinders and coils, all shapes resonating. Sequences rising and falling, fingers, everywhere fingers. The warm brush of lungs. Creaking of buttocks on chairs, slight releases of air, stomachs against belts, clasps and buckles, skirts rustling, paper finely shifting. Dry skin on palms worn down and rubbing together. Bells, diaphragms, stools, rib cages, all bones in concert, felt and leather above and beyond.

I shift in my seat. The desire to make things endlessly work has been my engine of action. I have been at war for so long. Failure is my best release. I am a gargoyle carved in stone: blasé, flippant, desolate. I do the things that are given to me to do: eat a bacon sandwich, drink a coffee, sit close and listen. One. Two. One. Two. In. Out. In. Out. I love being in position here. It is perfectly correct. This is where I should be. But I want him to stay with me. *Stay, just stay awhile longer.*

When we are alone, my voice sounds hollow as I talk to him while he sleeps. We have had the narrowest sliver of time, one pewter-coloured winter day, perhaps one and a half, of Tom being awake without words to speak at all. *Yes* and *No* have gone. And what happened? Our routes remained open. Language splits, folds, diversifies again and becomes a repertoire of homemade sighs and groans. We are in the versatile region of tone and touch and pitch mapped by light pressure to the skin or a hand circling the face.

Now, sleep is here. Sleep. No *Yes* and no *No*. No *Ah*, and no *Oh God*. *Eggsaaactly*, with such a long, drawn-out exaggerated *aaaaa*, went a while ago. It doesn't matter. We are gone into the grain, the sub-grain. Here *Yes* and *No* are the same.

I sound unnatural and false, like someone who is unsure to whom they are speaking and doesn't know how they should be addressed. I have the embarrassment of talking to myself lest I am not really talking to myself, lest I am *heard*. Sorry. I cannot make my sentences work. They tail off. This is a dry run. A premonition of what it will sound like when my main hearer is gone. I have lost the second consciousness that powers mine. Lost my sounding board, my echo, my check, my stop and finisher. I am down to one.

Tom said a corpse is potentially a comic creature. It is both active and passive object, an unstable hybrid of person and thing. What of the comedy of a man sleeping over three days and counting? It is so companionable this breathing, I wouldn't mind if it would only continue. In. Out. In. Out. My thoughts run on. Maybe we could live around it. We could manage. I would move in here permanently. It's a lovely room. Ev could grow up and become a teenager whizzing in and out, bringing his friends round for company and to keep the noise levels up or just out of sheer curiosity to check out the sleeping dad, the man in the bed.

My eyes are greedy. They are attuned to all they can get but here is an intensity of seeing I don't recognise. I know the room by heart but it's not the room I look at. I have his face. What do I see? Indents at the base of each hair of the beard where they poke differentially through the skin, the stiff white ones and the grey. Then, the silky long brown and the black hairs of the head; the bruised little flesh mashed so tender under the eyes with the eyebrows above like awnings on display. Then, the fine pores of the cheek and the coarser pores of the nose. Then, the battered lashes at rest below the clear span of the forehead. Looking is familiar. I do not drop my gaze. I am used to looking, thinking, revisiting, looking again. For hours and hours, for days. This is what I do. But I have never looked this way.

Here are permanent fires. We are frenetic and at the same time stilled, without motion, in wait for the main event. All our energy is burnt up in the one spot. We do not mind or notice this. All the high points and markers, the excitements, the visits, the work, the excursions, the exhibition, Christmas, a birthday, New Year, all these are merging, rolling together softly under a blanket of wool stitched with our names. Today, as yesterday, there are no markers at all. There is one more marker to come.

3.17

The body mechanical is subject to failure. The chest rises and falls. In and out, up and down, breath and pump, opposites in motion, apart and together, fuelling each other, breaking down, pausing, stalling, false-starting, flooding, jagging, getting cold.

Everything I see and feel is incompatible. What to do: stop or keep going? Stop now, or go awhile? Will my mind clear sufficient to the event? Enough. What is my mind anyway? No good to be had in it, stuffed with nothings, irrelevancies. Preparation will never be sufficient. We both knew that long ago. There is not clarity enough. The event is here, but now it has come I see it is here for me only and not for us. Tom is already elsewhere, gone on his own sometime in the last days. He glided so delicately out, his absence so continuous with his presence, with us and without us, that I didn't catch the moment and immediately it happened it had already gone and was behind me. So. Just me.

I am in place when there is a click and a discreet hum. A grey electronic blind outside the window smoothes down like a fourth wall, obscuring the sky and closing us in the room. I watch it without blinking. What can it mean? Is it a cue? A sign? Is it some anthropomorphic quirk of architecture that mimics the closing of an eye in homage, an electronic ritual of deference to the dying? Does the building *know*? How can it know? It is impossible. I must leave my pitch to find out. What does this mean?

It means nothing. It is a malfunction. The building is new. Its circuits are febrile and oversensitive and the vapid winter sun has activated all the sensors on the south-east face, making the blinds go up and down like semaphore all along its length. I find the operating button and raise it. Minutes later it eases down again. I raise it, furious now, jabbing with my finger. You see! The great bastard sun-star, the whole firmament contingent in opposition crowds in on me to distract and sap my attention. It will not leave us alone. It is just an endless interruption of small things. Leave us. Leave us please at last.

And now, something else: voices in a broil outside the door. Friends have arrived and I see them milling and crowding, their gestures blurred by the frosted glass. Among them is Ev. I have called them and not called them. It is the usual muddle. I stop the door open with my foot.

Ev is being handed over from one to another but I don't want to talk to them, only to him. I beckon and he zooms over. Without speaking I pull him in through the slit of the door. Now we are three. Three! How forbearing and bold he is. How gallantly he sets his face. His happiness is always at the ready to be pulled out of his belt and waved around like a plastic sword. He goes to the bed and pats Tom. He leans his head on Tom's arm. I salute him and release him and send him away. *Go now,* I hiss to the door. They must all leave, even he. *Stay, stay awhile*, I whisper to the bed. *Go away*, I speak to the door again. We have come so far I fear intrusion, someone bursting in on us with clumsy warm breath. *Go*. We want no vigils other than our own for each other. No waiting, no sitting, no row of mourners, no people slumped with faces set in readiness for news. I flick between the bed and the door willing them all away. My skin is live.

Finally they are gone. Everything happens anyway. Time is refreshing itself. I want this death to happen because it is the end and I will finally rest. I don't want it to happen because it is the beginning and I will finally understand. We are together on the bed. It is familiar. Like how we were.

Except no, the action is familiar but not the place. We have stopped being anywhere at all. We are way outside, out of culture, place, gender. I do not know where we are but I feel very sure of myself here. Time is refreshing itself, that's all. It is simple. Duration is the rope that drags and keeps us. Time is the fundament we have never left, so powerful is its agency and pull, so direct and strange. There is nowhere in the world like it.

How precious, I tell him, we are here and I am seeing you off. I am sending you. My hand is on his body. In and out. I am with you. In and out. My hand is on his neck seeking the place where it goes and finding it warm. I whisper something in time with his breath. My hand is in his hand. *Go*. I hum something, not anything. *Go*. I speak words, not anything. *Go*. I am not anything. *Go*. I am.

SECTION 4

4.1

10 January 2011

Dear Friends

Tom is dead.

He died yesterday, January 9th 2011, at 2.15 at Trinity Hospice.

With love

4.2

Two days after your death, in a dream you text me many times.

I read the first of them.

ME!

And so are the living comforted.

4.3

It was snowing on the day we buried you: small flakes, wide-spaced, tugged hard by the wind. Unplanned, we formed a circle around your grave and stood as the words went up. Your child and his friends were everywhere present in our procession, threading lightly through the lines of mourners. I scatter earth over you and so does he, fingers splayed back, palm flat. You have moved through us and now you are gone, leaving us standing. And so are the living comforted.